MW01115919

ATI TEAS® 7 STUDY GUIDE 2024

The One-Stop Solution for All Your TEAS® Study Needs. 3000 Questions and Answers to Pass the Exam on the First Try

By

Deborah Pence

✳ HERE IS YOU FREE GIFT!

👇 SCAN HERE TO DOWNLOAD IT

"100 Illustrated Questions on Text Comprehension"

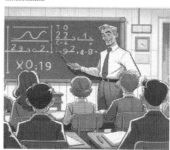

- Text Comprehension

- Use of Punctuation and Grammar

- 100 Multiple Choice Questions

- Table with Correct Answers and Explanations

Table of Contents

Introduction

Welcome to "ATI TEAS® 7 STUDY GUIDE 2024 - The One-Stop Solution for All Your TEAS® Study Needs", a comprehensive, meticulously crafted guide designed to help you pass the ATI TEAS® Exam on your very first attempt. This book is not just a study guide; it's a beacon of light on your journey to a successful career in nursing and healthcare.

Our guide is structured to mirror the actual ATI TEAS® Exam, ensuring you are thoroughly prepared for each section: Reading, Mathematics, Science, and English Language Usage. We've gone beyond the basics to provide an extensive array of resources, specifically tailored to cater to the ATI TEAS® 7th Edition, setting this guide apart as your indispensable companion for exam success.

What Makes This Guide Exceptional?

In-Depth Glossary of Key Terms: We understand that the foundation of any successful study plan lies in understanding the terminology. Our guide includes an in-depth explanatory glossary of key terms in the thematic areas under examination. With 103 terms of anatomy and biology, 100 terms in chemistry, 65 in mathematics, and 40 on the usage of language, this glossary is a goldmine of information, ensuring you grasp every concept with clarity.

3000 Practice Questions: Practice makes perfect, and with our guide, you get an endless supply of questions to hone your skills. This exhaustive collection of questions, split across scientific disciplines (1500), mathematics (500), and language usage (1000), is designed to test your knowledge and improve your understanding. This extensive collection is designed to challenge and expand your understanding, ensuring you are well-equipped to tackle any question the ATI TEAS® Exam throws your way.

Realistic Exam Simulations: To truly excel in the ATI TEAS® Exam, you need to experience the real thing. Our guide includes exam simulations, each featuring 170 questions, mirroring the actual exam's format and difficulty. Each question is accompanied by the correct answer and a detailed explanation, allowing you to understand not just the 'what', but the 'why' behind each answer.

This guide is meticulously structured, beginning with a thorough overview of the ATI TEAS® Exam, its significance, and how it is utilized in nursing school admissions. As you delve deeper, you will find chapters dedicated to each section of the exam, replete with strategies, tips, and in-depth discussions on various topics like Genotype and Phenotype, Macromolecules, and Scientific Reasoning.

We also understand the importance of psychological preparedness and test-taking strategies. Hence, we've included a dedicated section on preparing for test day, with effective stress management techniques, a test day checklist, and strategies for efficient test-taking.

In conclusion, "ATI TEAS® 7 STUDY GUIDE 2024" is more than just a study guide. It's a comprehensive learning experience, designed to provide you with the knowledge, practice, and confidence needed to excel in the ATI TEAS® Exam. Embrace this journey with us, and let's embark on a path to achieving your dreams in the world of healthcare.

Part I: Understanding the ATI TEAS® Exam

Chapter 1: Overview of the ATI TEAS® 7th Edition

1.1 Introduction to the ATI TEAS® Exam

<u>Purpose of the Exam</u>

As an aspiring healthcare professional on the path to a career in nursing, you will encounter a significant academic requirement known as the ATI TEAS® Exam. The Test of Essential Academic Skills (TEAS®) serves as a prerequisite for gaining admission to nursing schools. Comparable to the SAT in structure, the exam evaluates foundational competencies in Reading, Mathematics, Science, and English and Language Usage. Its purpose is to assess your aptitude for succeeding in a healthcare setting, rather than act as an impediment to your goals. Rest assured, this guide aims to provide comprehensive support throughout your preparation journey.

<u>Who administers the exam</u>

The ATI TEAS® Exam is conducted by Assessment Technologies Institute (ATI), an organization specializing in healthcare educational assessments. ATI has an extensive history in the field and collaborates with nursing schools and healthcare institutions to ensure the exam's relevancy and rigor. As such, the exam is not merely a collection of arbitrary questions; rather, it is a well-designed evaluation crafted by industry experts committed to your professional growth.

1.2 Evolution from Previous Editions

<u>What's New in the 7th Edition</u>

The ATI TEAS® Exam is continually updated to align with the evolving demands of modern nursing education. The 7th Edition embodies this adaptability and features updated question types and content areas that better reflect contemporary healthcare practices and educational requirements. This edition aims not merely to assess, but to thoroughly prepare you for future challenges in nursing.

Key Differences from Earlier Editions

If you are already familiar with the 6th Edition, you will notice several notable updates in the 7th Edition. Obsolete or less pertinent material has been purged, ensuring each question's immediate applicability to current nursing practices. Additionally, the exam's format has been refined to improve the user experience. While updates are significant, the exam's central objective remains consistent: to furnish a comprehensive evaluation designed to prepare you for a successful nursing career.

1.3 Importance of the ATI TEAS® in Various Nursing Programs - ADN vs. BSN vs. MSN Programs

ADN Programs

The Associate Degree in Nursing (ADN) offers a streamlined route to a career as a registered nurse. Prior to entering this program, the ATI TEAS® Exam is a required assessment tool that evaluates your foundational skills in science, math, and language. Consider this exam a critical milestone in your nursing career trajectory.

BSN Programs

For those targeting advanced or leadership roles within the nursing profession, the Bachelor of Science in Nursing (BSN) program is the optimal choice. Admission to these programs also hinges on your performance in the ATI TEAS®, which gauges your capacity to cope with a more rigorous academic curriculum.

MSN Programs

Lastly, the Master of Science in Nursing (MSN) is tailored for individuals aspiring to specialized roles such as Nurse Practitioner or Clinical Nurse Specialist. While the ATI TEAS® is generally not a requirement at this advanced level, the foundational skills acquired during prior preparations will undoubtedly prove beneficial.

Chapter 2: The Significance of the ATI TEAS® in Nursing School Admission

2.1 Role in Admission Decisions

Influence in Admission Criteria

If you are considering a career in nursing, the importance of the ATI TEAS® exam in your journey cannot be overstated. This examination plays a pivotal role in most nursing school admission processes, often accounting for 20% to 60% of the total admission score. Far from being a mere formality, the ATI TEAS® serves as a cornerstone of your application.

The examination is comprehensive, evaluating your skills in reading, mathematics, science, and English language usage. It serves as an indicator of your academic preparedness for the demanding coursework and clinical experiences that a nursing program entails. Excelling in the ATI TEAS® not only fulfills a requirement but also distinguishes you as a strong candidate for nursing school admission.

Typical Cut-off Scores

In terms of specific scores to aim for, the requirements can vary between institutions. However, most schools establish a minimum cut-off score, often ranging between 60% and 80%. This cut-off is not arbitrarily set; it is meticulously calibrated to ensure that incoming students possess the foundational knowledge necessary for success in a nursing program. While meeting the minimum score is vital, exceeding it can provide you with a competitive edge. Many schools employ a point-based admission system, where higher TEAS® scores can result in a more favorable consideration.

2.2 How Schools Use ATI TEAS® Scores

Program Placement

Upon receiving your ATI TEAS® scores, the next step is to understand how these results influence your academic path. Schools use these scores as key factors in determining program placement. High scores could potentially fast-track you into more advanced programs, positioning you for a more expedited educational journey. Conversely, lower scores may lead to placement in foundational or bridge programs designed to enhance your academic skills.

Your ATI TEAS® score serves as more than a mere numerical representation of your capabilities; it acts as a strategic tool to align you with the nursing program where you are most likely to succeed.

Scholarship Opportunities

Financial considerations also come into play, as your ATI TEAS® score can be instrumental in securing scholarships. Both educational institutions and external organizations offer academic merit-based scholarships. A high score on the ATI TEAS® can qualify you for these financial awards, substantially reducing your tuition costs. Even if your score does not place you in the highest percentile, various scholarships have a range of qualifying scores. Each point earned on the ATI TEAS® could potentially translate into financial aid, easing your pathway to becoming a healthcare professional.

Chapter 3: Structure and Format of the ATI TEAS® Examination

3.1 Section-wise Breakdown: Reading, Mathematics, Science, and English and Language Usage

Understanding the structural components of the ATI TEAS® exam is critical for effective preparation. The examination consists of four primary sections: Reading, Mathematics, Science, and English and Language Usage. Each section is designed to assess specific skills and knowledge essential for nursing school.

Reading

The Reading section has a duration of 55 minutes and comprises 45 questions. These questions are categorized into three domains: Key Ideas & Details, Craft & Structure, and Integration of Knowledge & Ideas. Topics range from summarizing texts to interpreting graphical data.

Mathematics

In the Mathematics section, you will have 57 minutes to answer 38 questions. These questions fall under two main categories: Numbers & Algebra and Measurement & Data. Skills evaluated include, but are not limited to, fraction conversion, equation solving, and data interpretation.

Science

The Science section offers 60 minutes to complete 50 questions. Areas covered include Human Anatomy

& Physiology, Biology, Chemistry, and Scientific Reasoning. This section will test your knowledge on a variety of scientific concepts, from cellular biology to chemical interactions.

<u>English and Language Usage</u>

The English and Language Usage section allocates 37 minutes for 37 questions, focusing on three primary areas: Conventions of Standard English, Knowledge of Language, and Vocabulary Application in Writing. Tasks may include sentence correction, language evaluation, and paragraph structuring.

3.2 Types of Questions - Multiple Choice, Fill-in-the-Blank, etc.

The ATI TEAS® exam utilizes diverse question formats to comprehensively evaluate your skills. Multiple-choice questions constitute a significant portion of the exam, but other types such as fill-in-the-blank and hotspot questions are also included.

Multiple Choice: Each question is accompanied by four possible answers, of which only one is correct. It is crucial to read all options carefully.

Fill-in-the-Blank: These questions require you to provide the answer without multiple-choice options, assessing your grasp and recall of the material.

Hotspot Questions: These questions present you with a diagram or image, and you are tasked with identifying specific areas. These are particularly prevalent in the Science section.

3.3 Time Allotment for Each Section

Effective time management is crucial for a successful ATI TEAS® experience. Each section comes with a designated time limit, and understanding these limits should form an integral part of your preparation strategy.

Reading: Allotted 55 minutes.

Mathematics: Allotted 57 minutes.

Science: Allotted 60 minutes.

English and Language Usage: Allotted 37 minutes.

3.4 Navigation and User Interface on Test Day

On the day of the exam, you will encounter a user interface designed for clarity and formality. Key features include:

Next and Previous Buttons: These allow for question navigation. It is advisable to answer each question before progressing.

Flag for Review: For challenging questions, you have the option to flag them for later review. Make certain to revisit these before your time concludes.

Timer: A visible timer assists in keeping track of remaining time, serving as an essential pacing tool.

Submit Button: Once activated, your answers are finalized. Ensure you review your responses meticulously before submission.

A thorough understanding of the question types, time allocation, and user interface is vital for optimal performance on the ATI TEAS® exam. Adequate preparation in these areas will significantly enhance your chances of success.

Chapter 4: Scoring and Interpretation

4.1 Scoring Methodology - Raw Score vs. Scaled Score

The evaluation phase, commonly known as scoring, is the crucial step that quantifies your performance on the ATI TEAS® exam. To comprehend the intricate process, it is essential to differentiate between Raw Scores and Scaled Scores. A Raw Score represents the total number of questions you have answered correctly. However, this score undergoes a transformation to generate the Scaled Score, which serves as the standardized measure for reporting.

The purpose of the Scaled Score is to ensure uniformity and comparability across varying test forms. The score ranges from 100 to 150, with an average generally around 120. This transformed score is employed by educational institutions for admissions.

You may ask how this Scaled Score is derived. The answer lies in a statistical process termed 'equating,' designed to adjust for the difficulty level of different test forms. Thus, the equating process ensures that Scaled Scores reflect the same level of proficiency, regardless of the test form taken.

Understanding the difference between Raw and Scaled Scores is crucial for accurate interpretation of your results. Raw Scores provide a basic understanding of your performance during practice, but the Scaled Score is what ultimately counts.

The ATI TEAS® employs a dual-phase scoring methodology involving the conversion of Raw Scores into Scaled Scores through equating, thereby ensuring fairness and comparability.

4.2   Interpretation of Scores

Having received your Scaled Score, you may be curious about its implications. First, it's vital to understand what constitutes a 'Good Score.' A Scaled Score can range between 100 and 150, with different educational programs holding varied expectations. While a score of 120 is generally considered good, programs might have specific cut-off scores depending on their competitiveness. Apart from the Scaled Score, your percentile rank offers another perspective by indicating your performance relative to other test-takers.

Understanding your Scaled Score and percentile rank equips you with valuable insights for your educational journey. These metrics serve as a comprehensive indicator of your strengths and areas for improvement.

4.3   Retrieval and Distribution of Scores

Upon completion of the exam, you'll receive an email notification directing you to access your scores via your ATI account. Once accessed, it's advisable to download a PDF for record-keeping. Distributing these scores to your prospective schools typically involves sending them electronically through the ATI platform, although specific requirements may vary. Be attentive to details to ensure successful transmission of scores.

4.4 Retaking the Exam: Rules and Recommendations

Should you contemplate retaking the exam, it's essential to familiarize yourself with the regulations set forth by the educational institutions of interest, which may include mandatory waiting periods. Recommended preparatory steps include a thorough review of your previous score report to identify weaknesses and comprehensive practice exams to enhance your comfort level with the test format.

In summary, strategic planning, rigorous practice, and a positive mindset are indispensable for retaking the ATI TEAS® exam. With proper preparation, you are well-positioned to improve your score and achieve your educational goals.

Part II: Preparing for the Exam

Chapter 5: Study Strategies and Tips for the ATI TEAS® Exam

5.1 Techniques for Distinct Exam Segments

Having gained an understanding of the intricacies of the ATI TEAS® exam, the next objective is to delve into strategies for excelling in each specific section. This chapter aims to provide a comprehensive guide to methods that can be employed for mastering the test.

Strategies for Reading Comprehension

Contrary to common belief, the Reading section is not merely an evaluation of one's ability to read, but also encompasses understanding, analysis, and interpretation of the text. To prepare effectively, one is encouraged to engage in active reading, involving marking essential points, notetaking, and posing questions during reading. This practice enhances retention and comprehension of the material.

Additionally, honing your summarization skills can be invaluable. After perusing a passage, attempt to encapsulate it in your own words, thereby gaining a clear understanding of both the main points and the supporting details. Don't neglect vocabulary either; unfamiliar terms should be looked up and understood as they can significantly impact your comprehension.

Techniques for Science Study

The Science section extends beyond mere high school biology to offer a broad overview that includes anatomy, physiology, and life sciences. First and foremost, organization is key. Draft a structured study schedule that earmarks time for various topics. Last-minute cramming is highly discouraged.

Use flashcards to facilitate the memorization of scientific terms and theories. Alongside, consider using visualization tools such as diagrams, flowcharts, or educational videos for better understanding of complicated processes. If you prefer a tactile approach to learning, online simulations or hands-on experiments are advisable.

Mathematical Problem-Solving Methods

For those who find mathematics daunting, specialized strategies can help overcome anxieties and enhance your score. Identify the types of problems you will face—ranging from algebraic equations to data interpretation and measurements—to tailor your study approach accordingly.

Persistent practice is essential. Solve a variety of problems, including those that challenge your critical thinking skills. Understand that errors are a part of the learning curve; if mistakes are made, take time to analyze them in order to avoid repetition in the future. When faced with complex problems, breaking them down into manageable steps is highly beneficial.

5.2   The Role of Practice and Review

Shifting focus, it's essential to examine the role of practice tests and reviews in refining your exam performance. Far from being mere supplementary tools, they constitute the foundation for mastering the ATI TEAS® exam.

The Significance of Practice Tests

Practice tests serve as a rehearsal, helping you manage essential resources such as time, energy, and focus. They allow you to experiment with various strategies for time management and question answering, thereby acclimating you to exam conditions.

Analyzing Mistakes and Weak Areas

Post-test analysis enables a comprehensive review of your performance. It is not simply a matter of tallying scores but involves dissecting your strategic approach. Assess how time was allocated across sections and whether undue haste compromised the accuracy of answers.

Identify not just the challenging topics, but also specific question types that prove problematic. Once identified, modify your study sessions to transform these challenges into opportunities for improvement.

In summary, practice tests and review mechanisms work in tandem as invaluable tools for preparing you for the ATI TEAS® exam. Investing time in these will undoubtedly elevate your test performance and set you on the path toward a rewarding nursing career.

Chapter 6: Time Management Principles and Practices

6.1 Introduction to Time Management Concepts

Time management serves as the orchestrator of various life activities, much like a conductor ensures that each section of an orchestra contributes to a harmonious whole. Specifically, within the context of ATI TEAS® exam preparation, effective time management acts as the unseen director of your study regimen, practice assessments, and exam-day performance. In this chapter, we will discuss the critical importance of this skill and dispel prevalent myths that could impede your progress.

Significance in Exam Preparation

Firstly, let us explore the essential role that time management plays in successful exam preparation. Consider the analogy of a chef: the individual ingredients—study materials, practice tests, and review sessions—may be top-quality, but incorrect timing can lead to an unsatisfactory result. Analogously, superior study resources will be of limited use if time is not managed adeptly. Effective time management allows for the division of the overwhelming task of ATI TEAS® preparation into manageable, incremental segments, thereby enabling you to focus more on weaker areas while spending less time on topics you are already proficient in. This approach is not merely about the absorption of information; it aims for efficient and optimized learning. Proper time management can facilitate comprehensive coverage of material in a shorter period, leaving room for essential rest and mental rejuvenation.

Dispelling Time Management Myths

Let us address some common misconceptions regarding time management. Myth One: "I perform better under pressure, so planning is unnecessary." Contrary to this belief, last-minute pressures often compromise quality and retention of material. Additionally, the stress and anxiety accompanying this approach are generally counterproductive. Myth Two: "Time management restricts creativity by enforcing rigidity." This statement is a misconception; effective time management, in reality, establishes periods within which creative exploration can occur without the distraction of other obligations. Finally, the irony of Myth Three—"I don't have time for time management"—cannot be overstated. Investment in time management pays substantial dividends in the form of reduced study durations and increased efficiency.

6.2   Strategies for Effective Time Management

Having discussed the importance of time management, we shall now explore various approaches to implement it effectively. Since there is no universally applicable method, it is vital to select a strategy that aligns with your individual learning style.

The Pomodoro Technique

One popular method is the Pomodoro Technique, named after the tomato-shaped kitchen timer employed by its developer, Francesco Cirillo. This strategy involves working in focused bursts of 25 minutes, followed by a 5-minute break. After four such cycles, a longer break of 15-30 minutes is recommended. This technique capitalizes on the brain's natural capacity for maintaining concentration over shorter intervals, thus fostering productivity and sustained attention.

Time Blocking

Another effective strategy is Time Blocking, where each task or group of tasks is assigned a specific time slot within your daily schedule. This method eliminates decision paralysis often linked with open-ended to-do lists and enhances productivity by defining the scope of each study session.

Prioritization Methods

Lastly, the Eisenhower Matrix offers a prioritization framework, categorizing tasks based on their urgency and importance. It's a simple tool that helps you categorize tasks into four quadrants based on their urgency and importance. Tasks that are both urgent and important go in Quadrant 1 and should be tackled first. Tasks that are important but not urgent go in Quadrant 2 and can be scheduled for later. Quadrants 3 and 4 contain tasks that are either not important, not urgent, or neither, and should be delegated or eliminated.

6.3   Achieving a Balanced Life-Study Equation

While mastering time management techniques is crucial, it's imperative to remember that a balance between study and personal life is vital for overall well-being and sustained performance.

Study-Life Equilibrium Strategies

One core principle is the "Work Hard, Play Hard" philosophy. Dedication to exam preparation deserves commendation, but leisure and self-care activities should not be overlooked. Engaging in hobbies, social interactions, and physical activities provides mental refreshment and a renewed perspective upon return to studying.

The Role of a Support Network

Communication is the cornerstone of a balanced life. Informing your social circle about your study commitments allows for mutual understanding and support, thus facilitating a harmonious balance between personal and academic life.

Importance of Intentional Breaks

Scheduled breaks during study sessions and longer leisure activities contribute to emotional and intellectual well-being. Furthermore, daily rituals that bring joy serve as minor rewards and enrich the overall quality of life.

In conclusion, achieving a balanced life-study dynamic involves more than sheer academic focus; it requires a holistic approach that also factors in mental and emotional well-being. Successfully navigating the journey to excel in the ATI TEAS® examination involves stamina, strategy, and the wisdom to appreciate the broader landscape of life.

Chapter 7: Formulating an Effective Study Plan

7.1   Introduction to Study Plans

Having mastered time-management skills and achieved a balance between life and academic pursuits, you are well on your way to educational success. However, the crux of this balance lies in the implementation of a comprehensive study plan, which serves as your navigational chart to ATI TEAS® success. This chapter aims to elucidate the importance of a study plan and delineate the elements that contribute to its effectiveness.

The Imperative of a Study Plan

Navigating your ATI TEAS® preparation without a study plan is akin to embarking on a journey without a map. A study plan is not a mere timetable; it is a strategic document that delineates your objectives, timelines, and required resources. This personalized blueprint serves as your guide through the extensive syllabus, ensuring that you stay on course.

A study plan fosters discipline and accountability, reducing the tendency to procrastinate or veer off track. A well-conceived strategy motivates adherence, acting as a cognitive coach that compels you to attain your academic objectives. Additionally, a study plan facilitates the assessment of your progress, allowing you to discern accomplishments and areas requiring further attention, thus making your study sessions both productive and efficient.

Elements of an Effective Study Plan

An exemplary study plan is characterized by its realism, comprehensiveness, adaptability, and resourcefulness. Setting unreasonable expectations, such as dedicating twelve hours a day to studying, is neither feasible nor healthy. Your plan should be congruent with your lifestyle, commitments, and stamina.

In terms of scope, the study plan must encompass all subjects and topics appearing in the ATI TEAS® examination. Decompose the syllabus into digestible segments and designate specific time intervals for each. This approach prevents last-minute cramming and ensures that no subject is overlooked.

Flexibility is also vital. Unanticipated events are inevitable; hence, your study plan should incorporate buffer days to accommodate these occurrences or topics that necessitate additional time for mastery.

Incorporate periodic review sessions and practice tests, which act as milestones for evaluating your understanding and retention of the material. Think of these as pit stops that allow you to refuel and recalibrate your strategy.

Lastly, enumerate the resources you will utilize, including textbooks, online courses, and other study aids. This preemptive measure negates the need to scramble for materials, allowing you to concentrate on the task at hand.

In summary, an effective study plan is realistic, all-encompassing, adaptable, and well-resourced. It is an indispensable tool in achieving ATI TEAS® success. Devote time to crafting one that aligns with your individual needs, and witness your preparation transform into a synchronized symphony of productivity. Your future self will undoubtedly express gratitude.

7.2   Constructing Your Study Plan

Convinced of the necessity for a study plan, you may wonder how to formulate one that transcends a mere checklist. Let's explore the details.

Establishing SMART Goals

Initiate your plan by setting SMART goals—Specific, Measurable, Achievable, Relevant, and Time-bound. These components are not jargon but are, in fact, the fundamental constituents of a functioning study plan. Be specific in your objectives; rather than stating, "I will study more," specify, "I will complete 30 practice questions on human anatomy every Tuesday." Make your goals quantifiable, achievable, pertinent to the ATI TEAS®, and time-sensitive.

Time Allocation for Each Exam Section

The ATI TEAS® is comprised of four primary sections: Reading, Mathematics, Science, and English and Language Usage. Each section requires a distinct skill set and, correspondingly, a varying allocation of your time. Begin by assessing your strengths and weaknesses. Designate more time to areas requiring improvement, but do not neglect your strong points. Balance is crucial; for example, if Science is a particular challenge, you may allocate three study sessions per week to it, contrasted with one for Reading.

In conclusion, constructing a study plan is akin to developing a customized blueprint for success. With SMART goals and judicious time allocation, you will be well-prepared to excel in the ATI TEAS® examination. Equip yourself with your planner, and commence your journey toward academic achievement.

Part III: Reading Section

Chapter 8: Examination of Key Concepts and Details

8.1 Introduction to Key Concepts and Details

Congratulations on progressing to the Reading Section of the ATI TEAS® exam. This critical segment evaluates your capability to process and interpret written information effectively. This chapter aims to provide an in-depth analysis of the core elements that constitute this section.

<u>Significance in Reading Comprehension</u>

Reading comprehension transcends the mere act of word recognition; it necessitates understanding the fundamental ideas and intricate details presented. In the context of the ATI TEAS® exam, possessing this skill is mandatory. The Reading Section is specifically engineered to gauge your ability to discern principal ideas, isolate specific details, and differentiate between pertinent and supplementary information. It is vital to recognize that these competencies are not merely test-oriented; they are essential attributes that you will require in healthcare settings where misinterpretations can lead to severe outcomes.

<u>Overview of Section Content</u>

The Reading Section will present a diversified selection of texts such as scientific articles, historical documents, and potentially, technical manuals. Expect questions that require you to identify a passage's main idea, locate particular details, and possibly even make inferences. You may also encounter items that assess your ability to distinguish between factual statements and opinions or identify the author's tone and intent.

In summary, this segment serves as a practical exercise designed to prepare you for the real-world challenges you will encounter in healthcare environments. It necessitates agility, attention to detail, and analytical thinking. Each question should be seen as an opportunity to demonstrate your readiness for a healthcare career. The Reading Section is not merely an evaluative hurdle but a preview of the critical skills you will employ professionally.

8.2 Types of Key Concepts

Explicit vs. Implicit Concepts

Let us delve into the types of key concepts you will encounter. First, we consider explicit and implicit concepts. Explicit concepts are straightforwardly presented within the text, requiring no additional interpretation. They serve as the foundational elements of comprehension. Implicit concepts, conversely, are subtly conveyed or suggested, necessitating analytical thinking for their discovery. In the realm of healthcare, understanding what is implicitly presented is often as crucial as what is explicitly stated.

Identifying Central Themes

Central themes represent the overarching message or lesson that a text aims to convey. In the ATI TEAS® Reading Section, questions may ask you to identify these central themes. This is not just an academic requirement but a skill with real-world applications. For instance, in nursing, you will have to integrate patient symptoms, historical data, and test results to diagnose the underlying health condition effectively.

8.3 Types of Details

Factual Details

Beginning with factual details, these are the unequivocal, objective pieces of information that underpin any text. In a healthcare context, such details are fundamental. For example, consider the statement: "The patient's blood pressure is 120/80, and they are taking 50mg of Metoprolol daily." Here, the blood pressure and medication dosage represent factual details.

Interpretive Details

Following factual details, we have interpretive details. These require discernment and are often deduced or inferred from the text. For example, an extended version of the previous statement might read: "The patient's blood pressure is 120/80, and they are taking 50mg of Metoprolol daily. They appear more relaxed and smile frequently." Here, the patient's emotional state represents an interpretive detail.

Both factual and interpretive details hold significance in healthcare. While factual details provide the objective groundwork, interpretive details offer insights into the patient's overall well-being, influencing a more holistic approach to care.

In conclusion, understanding both the types of details and key concepts is indispensable, not merely for test-taking but for your broader professional development. This dual focus will equip you with a comprehensive skill set, serving you effectively in your forthcoming nursing career.

Chapter 9: Topic Identification

9.1 Introduction to Topic Identification

Significance in Analyzing Texts

Welcome to the realm of topic identification, a foundational skill in reading comprehension. You may ask, "Why is this essential?" Identifying a topic acts as a preliminary framework for understanding the subsequent contents of a text. It serves as an initial guide, allowing you to forecast the types of information, arguments, and conclusions that may follow. Similar to recognizing a film as a thriller, expectations for suspense and plot development are naturally set. Recognizing the topic in a reading passage thus helps to engage your prior knowledge, focus your concentration, and deepen your interaction with the text.

Common Challenges

However, the task of identifying topics is not without its challenges. A frequent error is conflating the topic with the main idea. The topic represents the subject under discussion, whereas the main idea encompasses the author's particular point about that subject. Furthermore, there is the hazard of overcomplicating the topic. Occasionally, the subject matter is as straightforward as it initially appears, devoid of any hidden intricacies. Therefore, avoid needless complexity.

Additionally, the risk of hastily skimming and consequently missing the topic entirely should not be discounted. A failure to properly identify the topic could leave one adrift in a sea of ideas and verbiage. This is why it is imperative to take your time and be attentive to the text, as the topic is often manifest in the title, introductory sentences, or even dispersed throughout the text.

Are you prepared to master the art of topic identification? Armed with focus and a keen sense for detail, you will be well-equipped to sidestep these common pitfalls and immerse yourself in the enriching world of textual analysis.

9.2   Techniques for Identifying Topics

Skimming and Scanning Techniques

Now, let us delve into the mechanics of identifying topics. Initially, we address skimming and scanning, the core techniques for rapid reading. Skimming resembles an aerial overview of the text, capturing key elements without becoming ensnared in minutiae. This involves perusing headings, subheadings, and often the opening and closing sentences of paragraphs. Scanning, by contrast, operates as a focused search for particular terms, names, or phrases pertinent to the topic. Both skimming and scanning function most effectively when applied in tandem; skim for a general understanding and scan to refine it.

Contextual Clues

Additionally, contextual clues serve as invaluable aids in reading comprehension. These are surrounding words or phrases that clarify the meaning of an unfamiliar term or concept. For instance, if one encounters a sentence like, "The arid landscape indicated a lack of water," the term 'arid' directly correlates to the absence of water, thereby signaling the topic could pertain to water scarcity or desert ecosystems. Contextual clues can be definitions, examples, or even contrasting ideas.

9.3   Practical Exercises

Sample Texts

Theory is beneficial, but proficiency is achieved through practice. Sample texts serve as an ideal training ground, encapsulating a myriad of topics, styles, and complexities. To diversify your skills, select a range of subjects and levels of difficulty. Once you have your sample texts, employ your skimming and scanning techniques to discern the primary topics and subtopics.

Topic Identification Exercises

To further refine your skills, engage in topic identification exercises. These specialized drills often include a set of questions or prompts designed to assess your ability to identify the main topic, subtopics, and sometimes even the author's intent. For instance, you may encounter a text about coral reefs, followed by questions such as, "What is the primary topic?" or "Identify a subtopic presented in the third paragraph." These exercises require you to actively apply skimming, scanning, and contextual clue techniques.

The expertise in identifying topics extends beyond the academic sphere; it is an invaluable life skill. Whether you are reading a news article, academic paper, or social media post, the ability to swiftly identify the main topic renders you a more informed and competent reader.

Chapter 10: The Interplay of Main Ideas and Supporting Details

10.1 Introduction

The Role of Main Ideas in Reading Comprehension

Understanding the main idea is akin to possessing a navigational compass for a textual journey. It serves as the structural foundation that cohesively binds various elements of the content. Mastery of this concept enhances your reading efficiency, enabling you to dissect and assimilate diverse types of textual material.

Definitions and Contextual Illustrations

The main idea is the central thesis that the author aims to communicate, while supporting details are the subsidiary elements that bolster this central point. For instance, in a discourse concerning the health benefits of physical exercise, the main idea might be framed as, "Physical exercise contributes positively to overall health." This is further substantiated by supporting details such as "enhances cardiovascular functionality" or "facilitates weight management." As you engage in reading, bear these conceptual tools in mind; they are integral to your comprehension toolkit.

10.2 Methodologies for Identifying Main Ideas

Identification of Topic Sentences

A preliminary step in discerning the main idea involves the isolation of the topic sentence, a sentence which encapsulates the core theme of the entire paragraph or section. Comparable to a news headline, the topic sentence distills the essence of the subject matter. While frequently located at the beginning or end of a paragraph, it can also appear mid-section. The objective is to identify sentences that appear to be thematic overviews rather than specific details. For example, if a paragraph discusses the benefits of a balanced diet, the topic sentence might read, "A balanced diet is imperative for comprehensive well-being," thereby providing a thematic roadmap for the subsequent content.

Exclusion of Extraneous Information

Not every sentence within a paragraph serves to fortify the main idea. Some may provide ancillary support, while others might serve as interesting, yet non-essential, digressions. Your responsibility is to sift through the material, retaining only what is pertinent to the main idea. This skill, once refined, enables you to focus on the most salient aspects of the text, optimizing your reading process.

Pinpointing topic sentences and eliminating irrelevant content are invaluable techniques for identifying main ideas. Proficiency in these methods paves the way for heightened reading comprehension skills.

10.3 Methodologies for Identifying Supporting Details

Seeking Illustrative Examples and Justifications

After establishing the main idea, the subsequent task is to identify the details that corroborate it. Consider the main idea as a pivotal argument; the supporting details act as corroborative evidence. One rudimentary approach is to seek examples and logical justifications that lend credence to the main idea. For example, if the main idea posits that "Meditation enhances mental well-being," supporting details could encompass research studies demonstrating reduced stress levels among practitioners of meditation.

Recognizing Cause-and-Effect Relationships

An alternative methodology for identifying supporting details involves discerning cause-and-effect relationships within the text. Such details elucidate why the main idea holds true. For example, if the main idea states, "Global warming contributes to increasingly severe weather patterns," a supporting detail might draw a cause-and-effect relationship like, "Elevated global temperatures result in polar ice melt, which subsequently leads to rising sea levels and more frequent coastal storms."

In essence, the act of identifying supporting details resembles a form of textual detective work. Whether it's through illustrative examples that provide direct evidence or cause-and-effect relationships that offer a logical structure, these details are instrumental for a comprehensive understanding and validation of the main idea. Therefore, as you delve into complex articles or academic texts, keep these methodologies at the forefront of your analytical approach. They not only make your reading more efficient but also contribute to a more insightful understanding of the material.

Chapter 11: The Art of Making Inferences and Drawing Conclusions

11.1 Introduction to Inferences and Conclusions

Definitions and Distinctions

The skills of making inferences and drawing conclusions are integral components of advanced reading comprehension. Inferring entails making educated guesses based on available clues within a text, while drawing a conclusion is the process of synthesizing all the available evidence to arrive at a reasoned judgment. These are not mere academic terms; they are crucial skills that convert reading from a passive activity to an intellectually active one. These capabilities enable a deeper engagement with the text and facilitate a nuanced understanding of both explicit and implicit messages.

Significance in Reading Comprehension

The ability to make inferences and draw conclusions enriches your reading experience by making it an interactive process. These skills serve as invaluable tools for critical thinking, allowing for a nuanced understanding of not only what is explicitly stated but also what is implied or left unsaid. Therefore, when approaching any text, it is beneficial to ponder the possible inferences and conclusions that can be drawn to gain a more comprehensive understanding.

11.2 Techniques for Making Inferences

Utilizing Contextual Clues

When encountering ambiguous or complex sentences, context clues can serve as essential guides for interpretation. These are the adjacent words or phrases that can help clarify the intended meaning. Context clues provide valuable insights into the author's tone, mood, and intent, effectively serving as an analytical tool for deeper comprehension.

Interpreting Unstated Elements

The skill of reading between the lines allows you to elevate your inferential capabilities. Your own background knowledge and personal experiences become useful interpretive lenses. For example, certain non-verbal cues in a narrative, like a character slamming a door, can reveal emotional states such as anger or frustration. This level of interpretation goes beyond simple understanding and enters the realm of nuanced engagement with the text.

11.3 Techniques for Drawing Conclusions

Synthesizing Information

Synthesis is the culminating step in reading comprehension. It involves integrating various elements— facts, details, and inferences—to arrive at a coherent understanding of the text. This is akin to connecting disparate dots to see a bigger picture, thereby transforming you from a passive consumer of words to an active assembler of ideas.

Making Logical Deductions

Logical deduction is the application of critical thinking to arrive at a conclusion based on the presented evidence. It requires scrutinizing the available information and asking, "What are the logical implications?" For instance, if a character in a narrative is consistently secretive and suddenly inquires about bank vaults, one might reasonably conclude that something illicit is afoot. This process transcends mere comprehension; it engages the reader at a level that leads to new insights and perspectives.

Chapter 12: Advanced Strategies for Reading Comprehension

12.1 Introduction to Reading Comprehension Strategies

Significance in the ATI TEAS® Exam

As you prepare for the ATI TEAS® Exam, a critical milestone in your nursing career, the Reading Comprehension section should not be taken lightly. This section evaluates not only your reading skills but also your abilities to understand intricate texts, make inferences, and draw conclusions—all within a limited timeframe. The results in this area are pivotal for your overall examination score; thus, it is imperative to approach it with strategic preparation.

Overview of Effective Strategies

Techniques such as skimming, scanning, and using context clues are foundational for rapid comprehension. Furthermore, the skills of making inferences and summarizing are invaluable. These are not merely test-taking strategies; they are indispensable skills that will be applicable throughout your nursing profession.

12.2 Strategies Covered

SQ3R (Survey, Question, Read, Recite, Review)

The SQ3R strategy is a venerable and versatile method for effective reading. It comprises the following components:

- Survey: Initially, skim through the text to acquaint yourself with its structure, paying attention to headings, subheadings, and highlighted terms. This preliminary step offers a contextual framework.

- Question: Formulate questions based on your survey to prime your mind for active comprehension.

- Read: Proceed to read the text, ensuring you assimilate the information in relation to the questions you have raised.

- Recite: Pause after each section to internally recapitulate the key points, which aids in reinforcing the material.

- Review: After completing the text, revisit the primary ideas to confirm your understanding.

Active Reading

Active reading necessitates a dynamic interaction with the text. It involves questioning, relating, and even critiquing the material. Maintain a mental dialogue as you read, connecting new information to existing knowledge. Should any aspects of the text be unclear, pause to resolve the ambiguity. Pose questions such as, "What is the significance of this information?" or "How does this relate to the main argument?" Active reading enhances retention and cognitive engagement.

Note-taking and Highlighting

Effective note-taking and highlighting are not mere clerical tasks but thoughtful processes that augment comprehension.

- Note-taking: During reading, jot down salient points, primary arguments, and relevant terminology. Aim for conciseness; your notes should serve as an abbreviated yet comprehensive summary.

- Highlighting: Exercise discretion while highlighting by marking only critical elements. Indiscriminate highlighting can obfuscate key themes during subsequent reviews.

Both note-taking and highlighting act as additional layers of interaction with the text, strengthening your grasp of the material and providing a useful resource for future review.

In conclusion, whether you favor the time-tested SQ3R method, the depth of active reading, or the efficiency of judicious note-taking and highlighting, these strategies offer proven pathways to excel in the Reading Comprehension section of the ATI TEAS® Exam. Utilizing these methods will significantly enhance your reading proficiency and comprehension.

Chapter 13: Practice Questions and Detailed Answer Analysis

13.1 Types of Practice Questions

Multiple-Choice Questions

Multiple-choice questions are a staple of standardized assessments, including the ATI TEAS® Exam. These questions present a scenario alongside several options, of which only one is the optimal answer. While the structure may appear straightforward, the exam often incorporates questions with multiple plausible answers. Precision in reading both the questions and the provided choices is imperative. Begin by eliminating patently incorrect options, then critically assess the remaining answers. The objective is to select the most suitable answer, not merely a correct one.

True/False Questions

True/False questions offer a concise format, demanding prompt yet thoughtful responses. Despite the seeming simplicity of having a 50% chance of correctness, these questions are designed to evaluate your comprehension of essential principles. Examine the statement meticulously for qualifiers such as "always," "never," or "sometimes," which may serve as indicators for the veracity of the statement. When uncertain, rely on your most informed judgment, as it is often more accurate than you might initially perceive.

Fill-in-the-Blank Questions

Fill-in-the-blank questions present an opportunity for candidates to demonstrate their mastery of specific terms or concepts. With no multiple-choice options as a safety net, your knowledge is put squarely to the test. Consider the contextual cues provided in the sentence to identify the missing term. If the answer is not immediately apparent, apply logical reasoning to deduce the term that would render the sentence both complete and meaningful.

Each category of questions on the ATI TEAS® Exam possesses distinct attributes and challenges. Multiple-choice questions assess your discernment in selecting the optimal answer, true/false questions measure your grasp of fundamental concepts, and fill-in-the-blank questions evaluate your depth of knowledge. Comprehensive preparation involving all three types of questions is advisable for a holistic approach to test-taking.

13.2 Answer Analysis and Explanations

Detailed Answer Key

The answer key is an invaluable asset in test preparation, revealing not merely the correct choices but also offering insights into the exam's structural logic. Far from being a mere enumeration of answers, it serves as a comprehensive guide to the intellectual landscape of the ATI TEAS® Exam. Therefore, a thorough review of the answer key is highly recommended as part of your study regimen.

Explanations for Each Question

If the answer key provides the cartography of the test, the explanations for each question serve as interpretative guides. These analyses furnish a deeper understanding of why specific answers are deemed correct or incorrect. They elucidate the rationale behind each question and provide clues to the thought processes that lead to the correct answer. Consider these explanations as miniature tutorials that offer a granular look at the nuances of the test. They help identify common pitfalls, underscore key concepts, and offer strategic guidance for future similar questions.

To conclude, the detailed answer key and accompanying explanations collectively serve as a potent resource for mastering the ATI TEAS® Exam. Both should be meticulously reviewed to gain a nuanced understanding of the test's complexity and to refine your own test-taking acumen. Remember, identifying and understanding your errors is the preliminary step towards avoiding them in the future. Invest quality time in these resources for optimal preparation.

Part IV: Mathematics Section

Chapter 14: Arithmetic and Algebra

14.1 Introduction to Arithmetic and Algebra

Significance in the ATI TEAS® Exam

The ATI TEAS® Exam is an integral gateway to entering a nursing program. A predominant section of this examination focuses on Arithmetic and Algebra. One might question the emphasis on mathematical skills in a healthcare context. To elucidate, nurses frequently engage in activities such as dosage calculations, unit conversions, and data interpretation. An error, no matter how minuscule, can lead to severe repercussions. The ATI TEAS® Exam rigorously evaluates these proficiencies to ensure candidates are adequately equipped for their future roles. In essence, precise numerical skills can have a direct impact on patient outcomes.

Topics Overview

With an understanding of the importance, let us delve into the specifics of this segment of the exam. Candidates will navigate through a comprehensive range of subjects, from foundational arithmetic processes such as addition, subtraction, multiplication, and division to intricate algebraic methodologies like equation solving and expression handling. Moreover, concepts of fractions and decimals, which can be intricate, will be assessed. Nevertheless, with thorough preparation, these challenges can be adeptly managed.

The Imperative Nature of Arithmetic and Algebra Skills

At first glance, one might perceive these topics as relevant only for academic pursuits. However, the applicability of arithmetic and algebra transcends beyond the confines of the classroom. Everyday tasks, such as financial planning, determining optimal shopping deals, or even ascertaining the quickest travel route, employ these skills. In a healthcare setting, the significance is heightened. Essential responsibilities, from drug dosage computations to medical chart comprehension and research data analysis, rely on these mathematical foundations. Thus, arithmetic and algebra are not merely academic subjects but indispensable tools for both personal and professional endeavors."

14.2 Fundamental Arithmetic Concepts

Addition

Elementary Addition

Elementary addition stands as the initial mathematical operation most individuals encounter, providing a foundational base for advanced mathematical procedures. This operation amalgamates two numbers to yield a larger value. Fundamental to arithmetic, it manifests in daily scenarios ranging from tallying grocery items to computing total expenditures.

Carry-Over in Addition

An advanced facet of addition, the carry-over, becomes essential when the sum of digits in a particular column surpasses nine. In such instances, the surplus value transitions to the subsequent column. For instance, while adding 58 to 47, the summation of 8 and 7 amounts to 15. Here, 5 is recorded, and 1 is transitioned to the adjacent column, yielding the resultant 105. Mastery over this concept is pivotal for intricate computations and finds repeated applications, inclusive of the ATI TEAS® Exam and practical scenarios.

Subtraction

Elementary Subtraction

Subtraction, the antithesis of addition, deals with deducting a value from another. It identifies differences between quantities and holds relevance in various applications such as budget management and determining residual tasks.

Borrowing in Subtraction

For instances where direct subtraction isn't feasible due to a smaller digit, the borrowing technique comes into play. This involves taking a unit from the adjacent column to facilitate the subtraction. As an illustration, while subtracting 47 from 58, borrowing is employed to modify 58 to 48 and 18, enabling the subsequent subtraction. Adeptness in borrowing is crucial for intricate arithmetic problems, especially for examinations like the ATI TEAS®.

Multiplication

Multiplication Tables

These tables form the bedrock of multiplication. Serving as rudimentary tools for multiplication, they facilitate rapid calculations. For prospective nurses, revisiting these tables proves invaluable for the ATI TEAS® Exam and subsequent mathematical tasks in the profession.

Extended Multiplication

For multiplying larger numbers, extended multiplication is employed. This method decomposes numbers into individual digits, which are then multiplied systematically. Such processes are imperative for intricate calculations, particularly in healthcare where precision is paramount.

Division

Brief Division

Short division simplifies division for smaller numerals. Ideal for situations demanding swift calculations, it becomes especially pertinent in healthcare scenarios such as dosage determination.

Extended Division

For comprehensive number divisions, extended division is the method of choice. This meticulous process divides the dividend by the divisor to discern the quotient and manage potential remainders. This technique proves essential for intricate mathematical challenges, especially those encountered in healthcare.

Order of Operations

Navigating arithmetic requires adherence to a systematic order, often abbreviated as PEMDAS:

Parentheses: Anything encapsulated within parentheses is prioritized.

Exponents: Following parentheses, any existing exponents are addressed.

Multiplication and Division: Subsequent to exponents, multiplication and division operations are executed from left to right.

Addition and Subtraction: Concluding the sequence, addition and subtraction are executed from left to right.

This structured approach ensures accuracy in computations, akin to methodical steps in medical procedures. Proficiency in this order is not only vital for the ATI TEAS® Exam but also for precise healthcare calculations.

14.3 Fractions and Decimals

Fraction Simplification

Identifying the Greatest Common Divisor (GCD)

To initiate the simplification of a fraction, it's essential to determine the Greatest Common Divisor (GCD) of both the numerator and the denominator. The GCD represents the largest integer that can evenly divide both numbers. As an illustration, for the fraction 8/12, the GCD is 4. While there are advanced methods like the Euclidean algorithm to find the GCD, for smaller numbers, one can list out divisors and ascertain the most significant shared divisor.

Minimizing to the Simplest Form

Upon identifying the GCD, the fraction should be minimized to its simplest form. Achieving this necessitates dividing both the numerator and the denominator by the GCD. Taking 8/12 as an example, dividing both numbers by 4 results in 2/3, a fraction in its most elementary form.

Simplifying fractions is a fundamental skill, not just for examinations like the ATI TEAS® but also for practical applications, such as sharing meals or computing precise measurements in healthcare.

Conversion Between Fractions and Decimals

From Fraction to Decimal

Converting fractions to decimals essentially involves expressing the same value in a more universally comprehendible format. This conversion is realized by dividing the fraction's numerator by its denominator. Using 3/4 as a reference, dividing 3 by 4 provides a decimal, 0.75.

From Decimal to Fraction

The reverse conversion, turning decimals into fractions, is slightly more intricate. Consider the decimal

0.75. The initial step involves identifying the number of places after the decimal, which is two in this instance. Subsequently, the decimal is multiplied by 10 raised to the power equivalent to the number of decimal places, transforming 0.75 into 75. This number is then placed over 10 raised to the power equivalent to the decimal places, yielding 75/100. Upon simplification, the fraction 3/4 is obtained.

Proficiency in transitioning between fractions and decimals is invaluable, extending beyond academic evaluations like the ATI TEAS® Exam to practical real-world applications, such as finance calculations or culinary measurements. Mastery over these conversions enhances one's mathematical adaptability, a trait highly commendable in professions like nursing.

14.4 Foundations of Algebra

Linear Equations

Algebra functions as the mathematical framework where both numerical and symbolic entities work collaboratively, paving a systematic path towards understanding multifaceted mathematical relationships. One of the foundational components of algebra, especially pertinent to the ATI TEAS® Exam, is the technique of resolving linear equations.

Singular Step Equations

Such equations serve as the rudimentary units of algebra. Consider the equation $x + 5 = 10$. The method to unveil x involves applying the counter operation—here, subtraction. Deducting 5 from both sides elucidates $x = 5$. Though elementary in its nature, it's crucial to be proficient in this stage as it underpins advanced algebraic operations.

Multiple Step Equations

These equations demand a more nuanced approach. Taking the equation $2x + 3 =$ as a specimen, the primary objective is to isolate x. Begin by nullifying the constant from one side, which leaves $2x = 4$. A subsequent division by 2 renders $x = 2$. Mastery in such equations is analogous to mastering a complex dance sequence, requiring rhythm and practice.

Equations with variables on both sides

Such equations can be intricate and necessitate methodical operations. Observing $2x + 1 = x + 3$, the astute approach is to unify x on one side. Simplifying, the equation morphs into $x = 2$. The central strategy is to distill the equation to its simplest form prior to resolution.

Algebraic Expressions

Algebraic expressions function as structured representations of quantitative relationships. They articulate the intricate interplay between numeric and algebraic components.

Combination of Analogous Terms

To illustrate, consider the expression $3x + 5x + 7y$. Here, $3x$ and $5x$ are analogous terms. Their amalgamation produces $8x + 7y$. This pivotal step aids in distilling an expression, enhancing its tractability.

Distributive Principle

A cardinal rule in algebra, the distributive principle permits a term outside a parenthesis to be multiplied across terms within. For instance, in $5(x + y)$, the result is $5x + 5y$.

Factorization

A strategic operation, factorization dissects intricate expressions into simpler constituents. Essentially the antithesis of expansion, factorization discerns the core elements constituting an expression. For example, $x^2 - 4$ can be deconstructed into $(x + 2)(x - 2)$.

Algebraic Functions

Functions serve as the conduits that elucidate the interaction of algebraic variables.

Linear Functions

Linear functions, epitomized by the formula $y = mx + b$, are pivotal in numerous sectors, from economics to natural sciences. Here, m delineates the slope, and b signifies the y-intercept. Such functions predictably manifest as straight lines on a graph.

Quadratic Functions

Quadratic functions, however, introduce non-linearity. They're symbolized by $y = ax^2 + bx + c$. The graphical representation, a parabola, is either concave upward or downward. These functions find applicability in numerous domains, from predicting projectile trajectories to economic modeling.

In summation, the mastery of linear equations, algebraic expressions, and functions is quintessential, not merely for academic evaluations like the ATI TEAS® but for fostering a robust foundation for higher mathematical endeavors. Comprehensive understanding and persistent practice are the keys to unlocking the intricate world of algebra.

14.5 Summary and Key Takeaways

Having traversed the intricate terrains of arithmetic and algebra, it's apt to momentarily halt, assimilating the acquired knowledge and contemplating its profound implications. This chapter serves to encapsulate the pivotal takeaways, underlining their profound significance for the ATI TEAS® Exam and elucidating the subsequent avenues for your mathematical exploration.

Revisiting Arithmetic Foundations

We commenced our journey delving into the rudiments of arithmetic, the cornerstone of mathematical understanding. It's vital to perceive arithmetic beyond mere computation; it's an intricate tapestry elucidating interrelationships amongst numbers. Our exploration spanned from elementary addition and its intricacies, like carrying over, to the nuances of subtraction and the pivotal concept of borrowing. We further delineated multiplication, emphasizing the indispensable times tables and the art of long multiplication. Our discourse on division encompassed both its concise (short) and detailed (long) paradigms. An integral part of our journey was acquainting ourselves with the order of operations, a beacon guiding us through intricate computational mazes.

Retracing Steps through Algebra

Transitioning to algebra ushered us into a realm where numerical and symbolic elements coalesce harmoniously. Our focus began with deciphering linear equations, ranging from the rudimentary ones that necessitate mere isolation of variables to more convoluted equations juggling variables on both sides. Algebraic expressions were our next stop, where we honed skills from amalgamating analogous terms to adeptly deploying the distributive property and mastering factorization. Our expedition culminated in discerning algebraic functions, with special emphasis on linear and quadratic archetypes, elucidating their distinct traits and real-world relevancy.

Relevance for the ATI TEAS® Examination

The overarching question is: Why are these concepts paramount? The ATI TEAS® Exam meticulously evaluates adeptness in these realms. Anticipate questions that challenge you to resolve intricate equations, adeptly analyze graphical representations, and extrapolate predictions from furnished datasets. Both arithmetic and algebra stand as pillars for aspiring healthcare professionals. From precise dosage calculations to astute interpretation of medical data, these skills are invaluable. Therefore, proficiency in these domains transcends exam preparedness—it's about fortifying your foundation for a triumphant healthcare journey.

Charting the Future Study Path

As we ponder upon future endeavors, the mantra remains: relentless practice. Familiarity burgeons with consistent engagement. Contemplate undertaking specialized arithmetic and algebra diagnostic tests to pinpoint your strengths and potential areas warranting further reinforcement. Aim not merely for comprehension but for absolute mastery. Harness diverse resources, be it traditional textbooks, digital tutorials, or innovative educational platforms. Encountering hurdles? Seek guidance. Oftentimes, an alternative perspective can illuminate a seemingly insurmountable topic.

In essence, your accomplishments thus far are commendable. Yet, the essence of learning resonates in continual evolution. Forge ahead, immerse in incessant practice, and not only will you triumph in the ATI TEAS® Exam but also establish a robust pedestal for subsequent academic and professional pursuits.

Chapter 15: Advanced Data Interpretation Techniques

15.1 Preliminary Overview: Understanding Data Interpretation and the Multifaceted Data Queries

Embark on an enlightening exploration of data interpretation, a discipline pivotal to comprehending the nuanced stories that charts and graphs narrate. Being proficient in data interpretation isn't merely an academic prerequisite for the ATI TEAS® Exam; it's an imperative for those striving for excellence in healthcare, where data-driven insights can profoundly impact patient outcomes. Let's meticulously dissect the various genres of data-centric questions awaiting your scrutiny.

Classifications of Data Queries:

Data interpretation is a vast domain, presenting diverse types of challenges tailored to assess varying competencies. We shall segment them into the following subsets:

Bar Graphs: Fundamental to data interpretation, bar graphs juxtapose quantities across categories. Their orientation can be horizontal or vertical, often appearing in clusters for multidimensional data representation.

Line Graphs: Line graphs chronicle trends over time intervals, spotlighting the evolution of specific variables, thus facilitating the identification of patterns or anomalies.

Pie Charts: The quintessential tools for portraying proportions, pie charts vividly depict the relative significance of various categories within a cohesive whole.

Tabulated Data: Eschewing visual intricacies, tables present data in its pristine form, essential for extracting precise values or for juxtaposing distinct data metrics.

Hybrid Formats: Occasionally, data representation transcends singularity, amalgamating multiple formats. Here, synthesis of information across mediums becomes essential.

Descriptive Data Analysis: Herein, data is embedded within textual contexts, demanding not just comprehension but also analytical acumen.

Scientific Data Interpretation: Pertinent to the healthcare trajectory of the ATI TEAS®, expect datasets echoing laboratory outcomes or patient demographics. These demand familiarity with scientific lexicons and units.

The Imperativeness of Data Interpretation:

The rationale behind this emphasis on data interpretation is multifaceted. The ATI TEAS® Exam evaluates prowess in data assimilation, calculation, and inferential reasoning. Moreover, healthcare mandates an intrinsic understanding of charts, patient data, or research outcomes. Beyond mere observation, it's about insightful decision-making.

Strategy for ATI TEAS® Data Modules:

The ATI TEAS® Exam expects a nuanced understanding of data, underpinned by sharp analytical skills and meticulous attention to detail. Preparation should thus encompass thorough comprehension of diverse data types and enhancement of analytical prowess.

15.2 Reading Graphs and Charts

Understanding graphical representations is akin to decoding a sophisticated language. Each graph, whether a bar diagram, pie chart, or line plot, possesses its lexicon, calling for a nuanced interpretation approach.

Bar Graphs:

Bar graphs are ubiquitous in data representation due to their intuitive design. Their spatial orientation, either vertical or horizontal, provides clarity in data differentiation.

Interpretation Guide: Categories, often on the X-axis, are represented by bars, with their magnitude, often on the Y-axis, depicting the data metric. Emphasize the Y-axis scale and discern patterns or outliers amongst the bars. Remember, labels often conceal pivotal information.

Pie Charts:

The pictorial embodiment of data distribution, pie charts encapsulate relative proportions.

Interpretation Guide: The entirety symbolizes 100%, with each segment reflecting a part thereof. Scrutinize labels or legends for segment significance, and discern predominant or marginalized categories by slice size.

Line Graphs:

For longitudinal data representation, line graphs are unparalleled, showcasing trends over intervals.

Interpretation Guide: Usually, the X-axis reflects time, with the Y-axis mirroring the monitored variable. Discern peaks, troughs, and stability periods. Multi-line graphs necessitate legend consultation for variable differentiation.

15.3 Tables and Other Data Formats

Despite their austere appearance, tables are repositories of raw data, offering insights without visual embellishments. Among tables, Frequency Tables and Cross-Tabulations dominate.

Frequency Tables:

Elementary yet insightful, these tables proffer data distribution clarity.

Interpretation Guide: Typically bi-columnar, with categories and their occurrences, they might occasionally display percentages. Focus on prevalent and sparse categories and discern underlying patterns.

Cross-Tabulations:

Complex and multidimensional, these tables reveal inter-category relationships.

Interpretation Guide: Rows and columns signify categories, and intersections unveil frequency. High or low intersections indicate category interplay intensity. Row and column aggregates offer supplementary insights.

In essence, while graphs and charts offer visual narratives, tables, in their starkness, provide undiluted data. Whether sifting through bar graphs, pie charts, or frequency tables, each tool, when adeptly wielded, can reveal profound insights. So, when confronted with these data tools, delve deep, allowing the data to unveil its tale. The mastery of this craft will not only elevate your ATI TEAS® score but also render you adept in any data-rich environment.

Chapter 16: Principles of Measurement

16.1 Foundational Overview: The Multifaceted Realm of Measurements

The ATI TEAS® Exam necessitates a profound comprehension of measurement. It extends beyond mere quantification, delving into contexts, units, and practical implications. Herein, we will expound upon the quintessential measurements you should acquaint yourself with.

Dimensions: Length, Width, and Height

While seemingly rudimentary, these dimensions are indispensable. They cater to varied scales—from spatial dimensions of infrastructure to microscopic cellular measurements. The exam might challenge you with unit conversions, such as inches to feet or centimeters to meters. It's imperative to refine your familiarity with conversion matrices.

Volume versus Capacity

Volume quantifies the space occupied by an entity, whereas capacity evaluates a container's maximal content holding potential. Recognizing the distinction and mastering the associated computation methodologies, be it the volume of geometric entities or the capacity of containers, is paramount.

Mass versus Weight

Weight, a product of gravitational force, varies with location, while mass, representing matter quantity, remains invariant. Although colloquially interchangeable, scientifically, and for the ATI TEAS® Exam, their distinctness is accentuated. Proficiency in unit conversions, say, from kilograms to pounds, is essential.

Temporal Measurements

Time, an abstract yet tangible entity, demands precision. The exam might encompass unit conversions or calculations associated with velocity or rate. Mastery over time measurements is non-negotiable.

Thermal Measurements

Temperature gauges the average kinetic vigor of constituent particles. Whether delineated in Fahrenheit, Celsius, or Kelvin, adeptness in unit inter-conversions and discernment of phase transition points is crucial.

To encapsulate, the ATI TEAS® Exam's measurement module mandates a holistic understanding, transcending rote learning. Beyond academic prowess, it's about deciphering the inherent significance of these measurements in diverse practical scenarios.

16.2 Systems of Measurement: A Comparative Study

Units of measurement provide structure and uniformity, facilitating unambiguous communication, especially in scientific and mathematical domains. The ATI TEAS® Exam underscores the significance of two predominant systems: The Metric and the Imperial.

Metric System

The Metric System, ubiquitously recognized, epitomizes simplicity and standardization. Predominantly base-10, it encompasses meters, liters, and grams as primary units. The inherent coherency facilitates effortless conversions. For the exam, proficiency in inter-conversions between units, ranging from millimeters to kilometers or milliliters to liters, is indispensable.

Imperial System

The Imperial System, predominantly US-centric, exhibits a unique set of units: inches, feet, yards, and miles for length; ounces to gallons for volume, and ounces to pounds for weight. Despite its intricacies compared to the Metric System, its prominence, especially in US daily parlance, cannot be understated. The exam necessitates fluency in unit conversions within this system.

In essence, both Metric and Imperial Systems, with their distinct units and conventions, demand adeptness. The ATI TEAS® Exam expects comprehensive fluency, mirroring real-world scenarios where measurements underpin accuracy in healthcare scenarios.

16.3 Geometry in Measurement

Geometry, often relegated to academic realms, finds profound applicability in pragmatic scenarios, including healthcare. Here, we delve into two primary facets: Area & Perimeter, and Volume & Surface Area.

Area and Perimeter

These metrics elucidate two-dimensional spaces. Area quantifies space occupation, while perimeter delineates space encirclement. For the exam, common geometrical entities, such as rectangles and circles, often feature. Practically, such measurements might aid in assessing a patient's wound expanse or infrastructure spatial dimensions.

Volume and Surface Area

Transitioning to the third dimension, volume and surface area gain prominence. Volume ascertains space occupation, while surface area gauges external coverage. The exam might focus on entities like cubes, prisms, and cylinders. In healthcare, be it dosage calculations or equipment sterilization, these measurements are invaluable.

In conclusion, geometrical measurements, while rooted in abstract concepts, have profound real-world implications. The ATI TEAS® Exam not only tests formulaic recall but also their pragmatic application. Thus, as aspirants and future healthcare professionals, cultivating a deep understanding will pave the way for both academic and professional excellence."

Part V: Science Section

Chapter 17: Fundamentals of Human Anatomy and Physiology

17.1 Introduction to Human Anatomy and Physiology

Relevance to the ATI TEAS® Exam

The discipline of Human Anatomy and Physiology is pivotal for aspirants entering the healthcare domain, and the ATI TEAS® Exam underscores this significance. A robust understanding of the human body's architectural design (anatomy) and its operational functionalities (physiology) is imperative for optimal patient care. The exam evaluates this expertise to ascertain the foundational competencies requisite for a healthcare curriculum. A superficial review of this subject would be inadvisable; it is integral to your prospective career in healthcare.

Schematic Outline of Topics

The ATI TEAS® Exam encompasses various systems encompassing the human organism—including cardiovascular, respiratory, digestive systems, and more. Cellular biology, organ systems, and tissue structures also fall within its purview. Furthermore, it delves into the intricate workings of the endocrine and nervous systems—the physiological orchestrators of the body. Proficiency demands not just rote memorization but a comprehensive understanding of the body's integrated functioning.

17.2 The Musculoskeletal Framework: An Overview of Bones, Musculature, and Joints

The musculoskeletal structure facilitates locomotion, allowing you to execute everyday activities. Functioning as the skeletal infrastructure, it provides structural integrity, facilitates mobility, and shields vital organs.

Osseous Structures

Bones, beyond their structural function, serve a gamut of roles—from safeguarding critical organs like the brain and heart to producing hematological cells within the marrow. Moreover, they serve as repositories for vital minerals, primarily calcium.

Muscular System

Muscles, the biomechanical engines, manifest in variants: skeletal, smooth, and cardiac. While skeletal muscles enable voluntary movements, smooth muscles operate autonomously within organs. The cardiac muscle, singularly, regulates cardiac functions. Muscular activity is characterized by contraction and relaxation dynamics.

Articulations

Joints, the pivotal connectors, integrate bones and muscular systems. Functioning akin to mechanical hinges, they facilitate varied movement modalities. Cartilage and synovial fluid cushion these joints, ensuring smooth articulation.

17.3 The Circulatory Nexus: Encompassing the Heart, Blood, and Vasculature

The circulatory system, a sophisticated conduit network, orchestrates the body's physiological transportation.

Cardiac Organ

Residing centrally within the thoracic cavity, the heart's quadri-chambered structure—comprising atria and ventricles—pumps blood, ensuring cellular sustenance. Its dualistic function entails oxygenated blood dissemination and deoxygenated blood recirculation.

Hematic Fluid

Blood, a dynamic transport medium, conveys oxygen, nutrients, and waste products. Constituted of erythrocytes, leukocytes, thrombocytes, and plasma, each component fulfills distinct functions.

Vascular System

The vascular pathways, comprising arteries, veins, and capillaries, ensure blood's cyclical flow. Arteries propel oxygen-rich blood, veins channel oxygen-depleted blood, while capillaries mediate the intermediary exchange.

17.4 The Respiratory System: Exploring Pulmonary Structures and Respiration Mechanics

Delving into the respiratory system, we unravel the intricate air distribution machinery facilitating vital gaseous exchange.

<u>Pulmonary Organs</u>

The lungs, housed within the rib cage, are intricate structures with alveolar sacs orchestrating oxygen-carbon dioxide exchange. A profound understanding of their anatomy and physiology is cardinal for diagnosing pulmonary ailments.

<u>Respiratory Dynamics</u>

Breathing, an orchestrated rhythm of inhalation and exhalation, is regulated by the diaphragm's and intercostal muscles' activities, mediated by the brain's respiratory center.

<u>Airway and Associated Elements</u>

The airway infrastructure—comprising nasal passages, mouth, pharynx, larynx, trachea, and bronchioles—guides inhaled air to the pulmonary chambers. Each segment plays a unique role in conditioning the inhaled air—humidifying, warming, and filtering—ensuring optimal lung function.

Conclusively, these physiological systems underpin our very existence. As you prepare for the ATI TEAS® Exam, immerse yourself in this vast realm of knowledge, for it lays the foundation for a successful healthcare trajectory.

Chapter 18: Life and Physical Sciences

18.1 Introduction to Life and Physical Sciences

<u>Significance within the ATI TEAS® Exam</u>

Transitioning from topics on anatomy and physiology, we now delve into the intricate spheres of life and physical sciences. This segment of the ATI TEAS® Exam holds paramount importance, evaluating a candidate's comprehension of everything from atomic structures to the expansive universe. It assesses your command over scientific tenets, the aptitude for scientific deduction, and the capability to interpret empirical data. Essentially, this segment gauges your scientific acumen, indispensable for those intending to join the healthcare domain. From dosage calculations to lab result analyses, a robust foundation in these sciences is pivotal for your prospective professional trajectory.

<u>Question Modalities</u>

Venturing further, the life and physical sciences segment is diverse, encompassing questions from various scientific domains. Expect queries on biology, focusing on cellular mechanics, genetic frameworks, and ecological systems. Chemistry will necessitate knowledge on elemental structures, compound formations, and chemical reactions. Physics will broach topics like force dynamics, energy configurations, and movement mechanics. Additionally, anticipate data interpretation tasks, necessitating the deciphering of graphs, tables, and charts for logical deductions. The array of questions includes multiple choice, true/false, and fill-in-the-blank formats, demanding versatility in approach.

Conclusively, the life and physical sciences segment of the ATI TEAS® Exam serves as a holistic assessment of your scientific acumen and rational reasoning. This section is indispensable for roles in healthcare necessitating a profound scientific grounding. It's imperative to understand that mere factual memorization won't suffice; it's the deeper comprehension and application in healthcare scenarios that truly matter.

18.2 Basic Chemistry Concepts - Elements, Compounds, and Mixtures

<u>Elements</u>

Starting our exploration, elements are quintessential building blocks of matter. In the cosmic framework, elements are the singular units underpinning everything. Defined as substances composed of only a singular atom type, elements resist further simplification via chemical processes. Analogous to primary colors, when judiciously combined, they manifest a spectrum of variations. Represented on the periodic table by distinct symbols, such as "H" for hydrogen or "O" for oxygen, understanding elements is fundamental to mastering chemical science.

<u>Compounds</u>

Proceeding, compounds are akin to orchestrations of multiple elements. They are substances birthed when multiple elements undergo chemical bonding in stipulated ratios. Water, comprising two hydrogen and one oxygen atom (H_2O), exemplifies a compound. Distinct from mixtures, in compounds, constituent elements transcend their individual characteristics, amalgamating into new identities. Compounds bear distinct chemical formulas denoting the constituent elements and their respective proportions.

Mixtures

Differing from compounds, mixtures are assemblies of multiple substances retaining their inherent properties. Envisage a fruit salad, where individual components maintain their distinct identities. Mixtures bifurcate into homogeneous (uniform composition like sugar in water) and heterogeneous categories (non-uniform composition like oil in water).

Significance and Broader Implications

Grasping these rudimentary chemical concepts is imperative for healthcare aspirants. Recognizing compounds like sodium chloride (NaCl) and its relevance as an electrolyte in physiological contexts is vital. Understanding the essence of mixtures aids in comprehending medication interactions. Preparing for the ATI TEAS® Exam demands more than mere memorization; it necessitates an intimate understanding of these principles and their intricate interactions, forming the bedrock of practical healthcare scenarios.

18.3 Physics Principles - Force, Motion, and Energy

Force

Embarking on our physics journey, force epitomizes the external impetus acting upon objects. It elucidates phenomena from vehicular propulsion to the act of lifting objects. In healthcare, grasping the nuances of force dynamics, like injection administration, is invaluable. Force classifications include contact forces (friction, tension) and non-contact forces (gravity, magnetism). Quantitatively, force is measured in Newtons, commemorating Sir Isaac Newton's monumental contributions.

Motion

Subsequently, motion delineates an object's positional evolution over time, encompassing aspects like trajectory modifications, acceleration, or deceleration. In domains like physical therapy, understanding joint and muscular motion is paramount. Diverse motion types exist, from linear to oscillatory, all governed by the seminal laws of motion.

Energy

Conclusively, energy signifies the capacity for work or effecting change, manifesting in myriad forms like kinetic, potential, or chemical. In healthcare, energy principles dictate myriad processes, from medication dynamics to the operational mechanics of diagnostic devices.

Relevance and Examination Implications

Understanding force, motion, and energy is pivotal, with practical implications in various medical procedures. For instance, in hemodynamics, force and motion principles elucidate blood pressure mechanics. Similarly, medical imaging modalities derive from precise energy dynamics. These concepts extend beyond theoretical realms, finding concrete applications in daily healthcare scenarios.

In summation, foundational physics principles are indispensable for the ATI TEAS® Exam. Beyond rote learning, it's essential to internalize these tenets, recognize their applications, and leverage this knowledge in tangible healthcare contexts, directly influencing patient care efficacy.

Chapter 19: Genotype and Phenotype

19.1 Introduction to Genotype and Phenotype—Conceptual Distinctions and Definitions

Definitions

Welcome to an in-depth exploration of genetics, where we examine the complex relationship between genotype and phenotype. To commence, the genotype refers to the genetic constitution of an individual, comprising a unique set of genes inherited from both parents. Analogous to an architectural blueprint, the genotype contains the comprehensive information required to construct and maintain the organism. Conversely, the phenotype represents the observable characteristics or traits of an individual, such as eye color, stature, and susceptibility to particular diseases. The phenotype can be thought of as the completed structure, built in accordance with the blueprint but also subject to environmental influences.

Divergences

One may naturally inquire, "Why doesn't the genotype invariably dictate the phenotype?" This question is quite astute. While the genotype provides the foundational framework, the phenotype is shaped by a plethora of factors including environmental conditions, lifestyle choices, and stochastic events. For instance, monozygotic twins, although possessing identical genotypes, may exhibit divergent phenotypes due to differing life experiences and choices. This explains the phenotypic variations among siblings despite a substantial sharing of genetic material.

Significance in Healthcare

The understanding of the genotype-phenotype relationship is paramount in healthcare. Specific genotypes can predispose individuals to particular medical conditions such as diabetes or cardiovascular diseases. Consequently, knowledge of one's genetic makeup can inform preventative actions and therapeutic interventions. Moreover, the burgeoning field of personalized medicine heavily relies on genotype understanding to customize treatments for individuals. This is not mere academic theory; it is practical knowledge with life-saving potential.

Implications for the ATI TEAS® Exam

This topic is particularly relevant for those preparing for the ATI TEAS® Exam, as the test assesses comprehension of these fundamental genetic principles. Expect questions that challenge you to distinguish between genotype and phenotype, or elucidate how environmental factors can modulate the phenotype. The exam is designed to gauge not merely your theoretical grasp but also your aptitude for practical application in healthcare contexts.

Summary

In conclusion, while genotype and phenotype are interrelated, they are distinct concepts of critical importance in both genetics and healthcare. The genotype serves as the genetic blueprint, and the phenotype is the manifest expression of those genes, shaped by a range of extrinsic factors. As you prepare for the ATI TEAS® Exam, it is crucial not only to memorize these terms but to comprehend their wider implications, particularly in healthcare settings. This knowledge forms an essential part of the skill set required for delivering effective, individualized healthcare.

19.2 Mendelian Genetics

Dominant and Recessive Traits

Mendelian Genetics serves as a cornerstone for understanding the mechanisms of trait inheritance. Named in honor of the pioneering scientist Gregor Mendel, this domain of genetics introduces the terms "dominant" and "recessive" to describe trait inheritance.

Dominant traits are those that take precedence over their recessive counterparts when both alleles are present. For instance, brown eyes are dominant over blue eyes, and the presence of even a single dominant allele will result in the manifestation of the dominant trait.

Recessive traits, by contrast, are only expressed when both alleles for that trait are recessive. Cystic fibrosis serves as an example of a recessive genetic disorder; it manifests only when the individual inherits the recessive gene from both parents.

The comprehension of dominant and recessive traits is vital, especially in medical contexts. It enables healthcare professionals to predict the probability of certain genetic conditions and provide genetic counseling to prospective parents.

Punnett Squares

Punnett Squares function as a valuable graphical tool to predict the outcomes of specific genetic crosses. Named after Reginald Punnett, these diagrams facilitate visual representation of how alleles from distinct parents may combine in their offspring.

Consider a trait regulated by a single gene with two alleles: one dominant (A) and one recessive (a). Utilizing a Punnett Square allows one to foresee the possible genotypes of the offspring, thereby aiding in healthcare decision-making, especially in the context of genetic counseling.

Summary of Mendelian Genetics

To summarize, Mendelian Genetics equips us with the foundational understanding of how traits are inherited through dominant and recessive alleles. Punnett Squares provide a visual method for anticipating these genetic outcomes. Both are indispensable tools in the healthcare sector, contributing to areas ranging from genetic counseling to personalized medicine. As you prepare for the ATI TEAS® Exam, it is essential not merely to memorize these terms but to grasp their broader applicability. After all, this knowledge is integral to a career where its daily implementation is expected.

Chapter 20: Non-Mendelian Inheritance

20.1 Introduction to Non-Mendelian Inheritance: An Overview of Topics

Having gained proficiency in Mendelian Genetics, one might feel reasonably well-versed in the subject matter. However, it is imperative to delve deeper into the more intricate realm of Non-Mendelian Inheritance, a critical area for understanding the complete spectrum of genetic diversity.

In Mendelian Genetics, principles such as dominant and recessive traits provide a framework for understanding inheritance patterns. Non-Mendelian Inheritance, however, explores the complexities that arise when these patterns are not strictly adhered to.

Topics Covered in Non-Mendelian Inheritance

Codominance

A situation in which both alleles for a gene are fully expressed. For instance, the AB blood type manifests both A and B antigens on the surface of red blood cells.

Incomplete Dominance

Here, neither allele is dominant, resulting in a composite of both traits. A cross between a red and a white-flowered plant may produce pink-flowered offspring.

Multiple Alleles

Occasionally, a gene may have more than two alleles, as is the case with blood type, which features A, B, and O alleles.

Polygenic Traits

These traits are controlled by multiple genes, each contributing to the overall phenotype. Examples include human height and skin color.

Sex-Linked Traits

These are traits tied to either the X or Y chromosome, such as hemophilia and color blindness, resulting in different inheritance patterns between males and females.

Epistasis

This occurs when the expression of one gene modifies or overrides that of another, as seen in certain breeds of Labrador Retrievers.

Environmental Factors

Occasionally, environmental conditions influence gene expression, as demonstrated by the Himalayan rabbit.

Mitochondrial Inheritance

Unlike most traits, which are inherited from both parents, mitochondrial traits are maternally inherited.

Genomic Imprinting

In some instances, genes are selectively activated or deactivated depending on their parental origin.

Importance of Understanding Non-Mendelian Inheritance

Proficiency in Non-Mendelian Inheritance is indispensable for individuals pursuing careers in healthcare or genetic research. The knowledge is instrumental in genetic counseling, personalized medicine, and epidemiology.

As you prepare for the ATI TEAS® Exam, it is advisable to thoroughly examine this chapter to not only enhance test performance but also deepen your understanding of the intricate genetic factors contributing to human diversity.

20.2 Incomplete Dominance: Traits in Blended Expression

Incomplete Dominance occurs when neither allele for a specific trait assumes dominance, leading to a phenotype that is a blend of both traits. For example, in a genetic cross involving red and white flowers, the resulting phenotype might be pink.

Real-World Examples

The snapdragon flower serves as a classic example of incomplete dominance. Offspring of a red and white snapdragon exhibit pink flowers. Another example can be found in human hair types, where a blend of straight and curly hair genes results in wavy hair.

<u>Importance of Understanding Incomplete Dominance</u>

Comprehending incomplete dominance is vital for multiple reasons, including its role in medical conditions and responses to medications. Such understanding is particularly relevant for healthcare professionals and researchers.

20.3 Codominance: Simultaneous Expression of Multiple Traits

Codominance is a genetic phenomenon where both alleles for a trait are equally dominant, allowing for a phenotype that fully expresses both traits. This would be akin to a situation where two exceptional talents are equally recognized.

Real-World Examples

AB blood type in humans is a paradigmatic example of codominance, as are certain breeds of chickens where black and white feather traits are both expressed in the offspring.

Importance of Understanding Codominance

The concept of codominance is integral to medical and scientific research, particularly in areas like blood transfusions and the study of certain diseases and conditions.

In summary, both incomplete dominance and codominance add layers of complexity to our understanding of genetics. Mastery of these topics is not only essential for academic success but also enriches our comprehension of the manifold ways in which traits are inherited.

Chapter 21: The Study of Macromolecules

21.1 Introduction to Macromolecules

Macromolecules constitute the foundational building blocks of biological systems, possessing intricate structures that serve pivotal roles in a myriad of biochemical processes. This chapter provides an in-depth exploration of these essential molecules, with particular focus on the types of questions that may appear on the ATI TEAS® Exam.

The Principal Categories of Macromolecules

Macromolecules are principally categorized into four classes: carbohydrates, proteins, lipids, and nucleic acids. Each class is characterized by distinct structural configurations and performs unique functions essential for biological existence. Carbohydrates serve as the primary energy source, proteins are the functional backbone of cellular structure and biological reactions, lipids act as energy reserves and comprise cellular membranes, while nucleic acids encode the genetic blueprints for all living organisms.

The Significance of Macromolecules

Comprehending the importance of macromolecules extends beyond academic pursuits and is vital for individuals in healthcare and scientific research disciplines. These macromolecules participate in virtually every biological function. For instance, insulin—a protein—regulates glucose levels in the blood, and DNA contains the essential genetic instructions for life.

Macromolecules and the ATI TEAS® Exam

Those preparing for the ATI TEAS® Exam should have a comprehensive understanding of macromolecules. The exam includes questions that assess knowledge of their classifications, functions, and locations within the body, along with their synthesis and decomposition processes.

The Intricacy and Elegance of Macromolecules

The complexities of these molecules are awe-inspiring. Consider proteins: they are constructed from amino acids and their functionalities are dictated by their highly complex and specific shapes. Even minor alterations in the amino acid sequence can drastically alter a protein's function.

In summation, macromolecules are the cornerstones of biological systems. They engage in numerous biological processes, making them an imperative area of study for healthcare and scientific professionals. As you prepare for the ATI TEAS® Exam, a thorough understanding of these molecules will provide not only a competitive advantage but also a profound insight into the biochemical processes that sustain life.

21.2 Carbohydrates

Structure and Function of Carbohydrates

Carbohydrates are biological molecules consisting of carbon, hydrogen, and oxygen atoms. They are primarily recognized for their role as an immediate energy source. However, carbohydrates also serve as structural components in some organisms and act as markers for cellular identification.

Types of Carbohydrates

There are three primary types of carbohydrates: monosaccharides, disaccharides, and polysaccharides. Monosaccharides, such as glucose, are the simplest form, while polysaccharides like starch and cellulose consist of numerous sugar molecules bonded together.

Carbohydrates in the ATI TEAS® Exam

Understanding carbohydrates' classifications, properties, and functions is imperative for the ATI TEAS® Exam. This includes recognizing the significance of carbohydrates in both human physiology and the broader ecosystem.

21.3 Lipids

Lipids are hydrophobic macromolecules primarily made up of fatty acids and glycerol. They are crucial for long-term energy storage, forming cellular membranes, and serving as signaling molecules.

Lipids can be categorized into several classes, including triglycerides, phospholipids, and steroids. Each class varies in structure and function, thereby contributing differently to biological systems.

For the ATI TEAS® Exam, it is essential to differentiate among various types of lipids and to understand their physiological roles. Topics may include lipid metabolism and the impact of lipids on cardiovascular health.

21.4 Proteins

Proteins are complex macromolecules made up of amino acids. They perform a myriad of functions, including serving as enzymes, structural components, and transporters.

Proteins are categorized based on function: enzymes, structural proteins, and signaling proteins, to name a few. Each type has a unique role in maintaining cellular and systemic homeostasis.

Proteins' diverse roles make them a key focus of the ATI TEAS® Exam. This may encompass questions about protein synthesis, folding, and the impact of mutations on protein function.

21.5 Nucleic Acids

Nucleic acids, namely DNA and RNA, are the macromolecules responsible for storing and transmitting genetic information. DNA serves as the long-term storage medium, while RNA plays roles in protein synthesis and gene regulation.

DNA and RNA are the two primary types of nucleic acids, differentiated by their sugar components and the nitrogenous bases they contain.

The ATI TEAS® Exam may feature questions on nucleic acid structure, replication, transcription, and translation, given their critical roles in genetics and cellular biology.

In summary, macromolecules—carbohydrates, lipids, proteins, and nucleic acids—are pivotal to biological systems. They not only perform distinct roles but also contribute to the intricate web of physiological processes that sustain life. Mastery of this topic is crucial for any healthcare or science-related field, making it a vital component for those preparing for the ATI TEAS® Exam.

Chapter 22: Microorganisms and Disease

22.1 Introduction to Microorganisms and Disease

Taxonomy of Microorganisms

Embark upon an exploration of the microscopic domain, a milieu abundant with diminutive life forms that elude unaided visual perception. This chapter will systematically elucidate the intricacies of microorganisms and their pathogenic potential, a subject of not merely academic interest but also pivotal for candidates preparing for the ATI TEAS® Exam.

Microorganisms, colloquially known as microbes, constitute a heterogeneous assemblage of minute life forms, including bacteria, viruses, fungi, protozoa, and algae. While certain microbes serve as etiological agents of diseases, a vast array of them are beneficial, fulfilling roles that are indispensable for sustaining life. For instance, gastrointestinal bacteria aid in digestion, while specific bacterial strains are employed in the production of pharmaceuticals and vaccines.

22.2 Bacteria and Viruses: Characteristics and Associated Pathologies

Bacterial Morphology and Function

Bacteria are unicellular prokaryotic entities, devoid of a membrane-bound nucleus. Their cellular architecture frequently serves as the locus of antibiotic activity. Bacteria can confer benefits—such as the Lactobacillus species utilized in dairy fermentations—or induce maladies, as exemplified by Escherichia coli, a causative agent of foodborne illnesses.

Pathologies Attributed to Bacterial Agents

Bacterial etiologies can manifest as a spectrum of conditions, ranging from benign afflictions like acne to severe, life-threatening infections such as bacterial meningitis. The standard therapeutic approach involves antibiotic administration, necessitating complete adherence to the prescribed regimen to mitigate the onset of antibiotic resistance.

Viral Structure and Pathogenicity

Viruses are acellular infectious particles that require host cellular machinery for replication. Their minimalistic structure typically comprises nucleic acid encased in a protein coat. Viruses are implicated in a plethora of conditions, from relatively benign respiratory infections to severe diseases like COVID-19.

Mastery of the morphological and functional distinctions between bacteria and viruses is indispensable for candidates preparing for the ATI TEAS® Exam. Anticipate queries that necessitate the identification of specific diseases as either bacterial or viral in origin, along with the corresponding therapeutic interventions.

22.3 Protozoa and Fungi: Biological Roles and Clinical Impact

Protozoan Characteristics

Protozoa are unicellular eukaryotic organisms, equipped with a well-defined nucleus and capable of locomotion via diverse modalities such as flagella, cilia, or pseudopods.

Pathologies Attributed to Protozoan Agents

Protozoa can induce diseases like malaria and amoebic dysentery. Typically endemic to tropical and subtropical zones, these diseases require prompt medical intervention for successful mitigation.

Fungal Morphology and Ecological Roles

Fungi comprise a diverse group of eukaryotic organisms that execute critical roles in nutrient cycling by decomposing organic matter.

Pathologies Attributed to Fungal Agents

Fungal organisms can cause a variety of diseases, collectively referred to as mycoses, ranging from superficial conditions like athlete's foot to systemic infections such as histoplasmosis.

A nuanced understanding of the biological roles and clinical impact of protozoa and fungi is critical for successful performance in the ATI TEAS® Exam. Anticipate questions that challenge your comprehension of the diseases these microorganisms can cause and their broader ecological roles.

Microorganisms, though minute, exert a profound influence on ecological systems and human health. A comprehensive understanding of their taxonomy, biology, and pathogenic potential is not only academically enriching but also essential for candidates preparing for the ATI TEAS® Exam. Therefore, whether you are utilizing antibacterial hand sanitizer or consuming probiotic yogurt, a cognizance of the microscopic realm will enhance your appreciation of its impact on human life.

Chapter 23: Scientific Reasoning

23.1 Introduction to Scientific Reasoning and Types of Questions

Welcome to the exploration of scientific reasoning, a critical skill not merely confined to professional scientists, but valuable for individuals aiming for thoughtful decision-making. In the context of the ATI TEAS® Exam, mastering the subtleties of scientific reasoning can provide a significant advantage. This section will elucidate the types of questions you might encounter and underscore the vital importance of this skill set.

Types of Questions: Classifications and Complexities

The ATI TEAS® Exam features a diverse array of questions aimed at gauging your aptitude in scientific reasoning. These questions span several categories:

Factual Questions: These questions assess your fundamental grasp of scientific principles. An example would be, "What is the atomic number of carbon?"

Application Questions: These necessitate applying your theoretical understanding to new or hypothetical scenarios, such as predicting the outcome of a chemical reaction based on given reactants.

Interpretation Questions: These demand that you decipher data or scientific charts, necessitating you to draw conclusions or make inferences.

Evaluation Questions: These are particularly challenging, requiring you to scrutinize the validity of scientific claims or experiments. For instance, you may need to identify limitations in a scientific study or evaluate the pertinence of certain evidence.

The Importance of Scientific Reasoning

You may question the necessity of scientific reasoning skills, especially for an exam geared toward healthcare professionals. However, scientific reasoning transcends mere factual knowledge. It is an analytic skill essential for problem-solving and evidence-based decision-making in healthcare, whether it involves patient diagnosis, data interpretation, or efficacy assessment of a treatment plan.

Scientific Reasoning in the Context of the ATI TEAS® Exam

Questions related to scientific reasoning on the ATI TEAS® Exam are crafted to measure your capacity for critical thought and problem-solving within a scientific framework. These abilities are not only pertinent for excelling in the examination but are foundational skills beneficial in any healthcare environment.

In sum, scientific reasoning is a multidimensional skill that transcends mere rote learning. It involves the application, interpretation, and evaluation of scientific data to make informed decisions. As you prepare for the ATI TEAS® Exam, focus on the application of knowledge, not just its acquisition. Proficiency in healthcare is not solely about possessing information but about utilizing it judiciously.

23.2 The Scientific Method: Steps and Practical Implications

The Scientific Method represents a structured framework that has underpinned scientific investigation for centuries. Contrary to being a mere procedural checklist, it serves as a holistic approach to problem-solving.

<u>Steps in the Scientific Method</u>

Observation: The genesis of any scientific inquiry, potentially as straightforward as noting a patient's symptoms in a healthcare setting.

Question: A formulated query based on observations, such as, "Why does this patient have a high fever?"

Hypothesis: An educated prediction or conjecture that serves as a tentative answer to the formulated question.

Experimentation: The stage where the hypothesis undergoes empirical testing, which may include clinical trials or a review of existing literature.

Data Collection: The aggregation of data to corroborate or refute the hypothesis.

Analysis: Data is scrutinized and interpreted to inform the study's outcome.

Conclusion: A determination is made regarding the validity of the hypothesis, necessitating either acceptance or revision.

<u>Application Beyond the Laboratory</u>

The Scientific Method is not confined to sterile labs filled with glassware and reagents. It finds extensive applicability in healthcare for diagnostics, treatment planning, and administrative decision-making. For example, if a particular treatment regime proves ineffective for a cohort of patients, healthcare professionals can employ the Scientific Method to investigate alternatives.

The exam will include questions to evaluate your understanding of the Scientific Method and its applicability in different contexts. These might involve identifying the sequence of steps, interpreting data, or assessing the soundness of conclusions based on provided data.

The Scientific Method is not merely an academic concept; it is an invaluable tool for evidence-based problem-solving in healthcare. As you prepare for the ATI TEAS® Exam, it is crucial not just to memorize the steps, but to comprehend their practical applicability.

23.3 Critical Thinking in Scientific Contexts

Critical thinking in the realm of science can be likened to a vital component that enhances the quality and outcome of scientific endeavors. It is not merely a process of data collection but involves a nuanced interpretation and assessment of the gathered information.

Data Analysis

This goes beyond numerical computation to include comprehensive review from multiple perspectives, pattern recognition, and critical questioning. In healthcare, this skill is vital for evaluating patient data to discern trends or the efficacy of treatments.

Drawing Conclusions

This is a pivotal stage where your critical thinking skills are indispensable. You must ascertain whether the data validates your hypothesis or suggests alternative conclusions. Additionally, recognizing the limitations of your data is essential, especially in healthcare where inaccurate conclusions can have serious consequences.

Critical Thinking on the ATI TEAS® Exam

The examination will assess your aptitude for critical thinking within a scientific context. This may involve questions that require you to interpret or evaluate data and draw meaningful conclusions based on it.

The Bigger Picture

Critical thinking is not just an exam-centric skill but a foundational attribute for any healthcare career.

Whether it involves patient diagnosis, treatment planning, or research, critical thinking aids in making evidence-based decisions. As you prepare for the ATI TEAS® Exam, consider honing your critical thinking skills through practice in data interpretation, hypothesis evaluation, and reasoned conclusion-making. These abilities will not only enhance your performance on the exam but will also prepare you for a more effective career in healthcare.

Part VI: English and Language Usage

Chapter 24: Fundamentals of Grammar and Sentence Structure

24.1 Introduction to Grammar and Sentence Structure

<u>Relevance to the ATI TEAS® Exam</u>

Grammar and sentence structure serve as foundational elements for the English and Language Usage section of the ATI TEAS® Exam. Mastery of these elements is essential for healthcare professionals to ensure clear and effective communication. Whether you are drafting medical records, explaining a diagnosis to a patient, or coordinating with fellow healthcare providers, your grammatical acuity is crucial. Communication errors could potentially lead to misunderstandings that may have severe repercussions in healthcare settings. Hence, mastering these elements is indispensable not only for exam success but also for competent healthcare practice.

<u>Topics Covered</u>

The ATI TEAS® Exam encompasses a variety of topics related to grammar and sentence structure, including but not limited to subject-verb agreement, verb tenses, modifiers, and different sentence types (e.g., declarative, interrogative). You will also explore punctuation mechanics, including the proper use of commas, semicolons, and apostrophes, as well as word usage differentiating commonly confused terms like 'affect' and 'effect' or 'their' and 'there'.

In summary, this exam section aims to evaluate your capacity for crafting and analyzing well-structured sentences and your understanding of the governing rules of written English. Therefore, as you prepare for the ATI TEAS® Exam, it is imperative to allocate sufficient focus to these foundational elements.

24.2 Subject-Verb Agreement: Principles and Illustrations

<u>Guidelines</u>

Subject-verb agreement forms a cornerstone of grammatically correct sentence construction. It requires that a subject and its corresponding verb must agree in number. While this principle may appear straightforward, it does possess nuanced exceptions. For instance, with the inclusion of phrases like "as well as," "along with," or "in addition to," the verb must agree with the primary subject. In the sentence "The doctor, along with the nurses, is arriving," the verb "is" concords with "doctor," not "nurses."

Examples

Here are some illustrative examples to elucidate this concept:

Singular Subject, Singular Verb: The nurse administers the medication.

Plural Subject, Plural Verb: The nurses administer the medication.

Compound Subject, Singular Verb: The nurse and the doctor are ready.

Principle of the First Subject: The patient, along with his family, is waiting.

Moreover, indefinite pronouns like "everyone," "nobody," and "somebody" are actually singular, despite their plural implications. Likewise, collective nouns like "team" or "staff" generally take a singular verb in American English but may take a plural verb in British English.

Special Considerations

Phrases denoting quantities, such as "a lot of," "a majority of," and "some of," may require a singular or plural verb depending on the noun they refer to. For example, "A lot of the medication was wasted" (singular) vs. "A lot of the pills were wasted" (plural).

24.3 Verb Tenses: Past, Present, and Future

Past Tense

The past tense contextualizes actions or states that have already occurred. In English, regular verbs typically adopt the "-ed" suffix to form the past tense, e.g., "The nurse administered the medication yesterday."

Present Tense

The present tense represents ongoing actions or general truths. For regular verbs, the present tense remains relatively simple: "The nurse administers the medication."

Future Tense

The future tense refers to actions or states that will occur. One can use "will" or "shall" in conjunction with the base form of the verb to indicate future actions, e.g., "The nurse will administer the medication tomorrow."

Consistency and Special Cases

Maintaining tense consistency is vital for readability and comprehension. Additionally, English incorporates perfect and continuous tenses to express different temporal nuances.

24.4 Modifiers: Adjectives and Adverbs

Adjectives

Adjectives embellish nouns by providing additional information about their characteristics. For example, "The skilled nurse gave the essential medication."

Adverbs

Adverbs modify verbs, adjectives, or other adverbs, answering questions like "how," "when," "where," and "to what extent," e.g., "The nurse quickly administered the medication."

Placement and Usage

The correct placement of modifiers is critical for conveying the intended meaning, as misplaced modifiers can lead to ambiguity. Similarly, the appropriate selection between adjectives and adverbs is vital for grammatical accuracy.

Modifiers enrich your sentences, offering greater clarity and precision. Therefore, mastering their appropriate usage is not just beneficial for scoring well on the ATI TEAS® Exam but also crucial for effective communication in your healthcare career.

Chapter 25: Vocabulary Enhancement

25.1 The Significance of Vocabulary in the ATI TEAS® Exam

Vocabulary extends beyond mere rote memorization of words; it is an integral component for comprehending questions, interpreting reading materials, and articulating your knowledge proficiently in the context of the ATI TEAS® Exam. This examination evaluates your facility with an extensive range of words, with an emphasis on terminology pertinent to healthcare environments. A well-developed vocabulary facilitates accurate navigation through intricate situations, comprehension of medical terms, and potentially enhances the quality of patient care in your future professional life.

<u>Subtopics to be Addressed</u>

In this chapter, we shall explore various dimensions of vocabulary that are requisite for excelling in the ATI TEAS® Exam. Topics will include common prefixes, suffixes, and root words frequently encountered in medical language, as well as synonyms, antonyms, and the subtle intricacies of word meanings in diverse contexts. Strategies for deducing the meanings of unfamiliar terms, a skill invaluable both within the scope of the examination and in real-world healthcare scenarios, will also be covered.

A comprehensive vocabulary encompasses more than individual words; it involves understanding various word forms, multiple meanings, and the nuanced differences between terms that may appear similar. For instance, distinguishing between the words "affect" and "effect" could be pivotal in a healthcare context, as their misuse could engender serious misunderstandings with genuine repercussions.

Moreover, the dynamic nature of vocabulary, particularly within the healthcare sector, necessitates continuous learning and adaptation. New terminologies and jargon are constantly introduced, requiring an ongoing commitment to vocabulary expansion that will not only help in passing exams but also contribute significantly to the quality of healthcare delivery.

In conclusion, vocabulary transcends the mere acquisition of words; it is about understanding their intricate meanings and applicabilities in a variety of contexts. Your ability to select the appropriate term for each situation ensures lucid and effective communication. As you prepare for the ATI TEAS® Exam, regard a rich vocabulary as one of your most valuable assets.

25.2 Key Terms for the ATI TEAS® Exam: Definitions and Applications

The ATI TEAS® Exam frequently features terms especially relevant to healthcare environments. Understanding these terms is essential for interpreting complex questions and medical documents. For example, the word "acute" commonly appears in medical discussions and refers to conditions that are severe but short-lived, contrasting with "chronic," which indicates long-lasting conditions. Terms like "benign" and "malignant" are crucial for comprehending medical reports, while understanding "contraindication" is vital for making informed decisions regarding patient treatment. Similarly, terms such as "empathy," "homeostasis," "osmosis," and "triage" hold significant implications in healthcare.

These terms are not merely items to memorize; they serve as the foundational building blocks for a more profound understanding of healthcare practices and protocols. Mastery of these terms will enhance your performance on the ATI TEAS® Exam and equip you for practical applications in your healthcare career.

25.3 Utilizing Context Clues for Deciphering Unfamiliar Terms

Encountering unfamiliar words in significant texts is an experience most readers share. While referring to a dictionary or conducting an internet search might be the immediate recourse, it is not always feasible, especially during examinations like the ATI TEAS®. Herein lies the importance of context clues—elements within the text that assist in deducing the unknown term's meaning. Various strategies include:

Synonym Clues: Sometimes, the text may offer a synonym that elucidates the unknown word's meaning.

Antonym Clues: The text might present an antonym, which could serve to clarify by contrast.

Definition Clues: Occasionally, the term's definition is explicitly stated within the sentence.

Example Clues: The text might list examples that help elucidate the unfamiliar term.

Inference Clues: In some cases, the term's meaning must be inferred from the surrounding context.

Punctuation Clues: Punctuation, such as commas or dashes, can offer hints toward the term's meaning.

Tone and Mood: The overall tone or mood of the text can also lend clues.

Acquiring the skill to utilize context clues effectively extends beyond preparing for the ATI TEAS® Exam; it is a lifelong skill applicable to any reading task. Therefore, the next time you come across an unfamiliar word, employ these strategies to decode its meaning. In doing so, you will not only broaden your vocabulary but also evolve into a more adept reader.

Chapter 26: Punctuation and Spelling Fundamentals

26.1 Introduction to Punctuation and Spelling

In the field of English language and linguistics, punctuation and spelling serve as integral components that provide clarity, coherence, and precision to written communication. Although they may appear less significant in relation to overarching grammatical rules and extensive vocabulary, their role in accurate and effective messaging is indispensable. This holds particularly true in contexts such as the ATI TEAS® Exam, where each syntactical detail may impact your overall score. This chapter aims to elucidate the importance of these elements and provide an overview of the topics under discussion.

Significance in the Context of the ATI TEAS® Exam

You may question the relevance of seemingly straightforward elements like punctuation and spelling in an exam designed to evaluate your suitability for healthcare programs. The answer lies in the critical importance of clear, precise communication within healthcare environments. Whether documenting patient records, interpreting medical data, or engaging in professional correspondence, lapses in punctuation or spelling can result in misinterpretations with potentially severe implications. Hence, a solid foundation in these basic components of the English language is deemed essential for aspiring healthcare professionals.

Overview of Topics

This chapter offers an in-depth examination of punctuation and spelling rules, facilitating thorough preparation for the ATI TEAS® Exam. Topics to be addressed include:

Punctuation Marks: A study of key punctuation marks such as periods, commas, semicolons, and quotation marks, along with guidelines for their correct application.

Rules of Capitalization: Though not a form of punctuation per se, appropriate capitalization enhances readability and clarity.

Common Spelling Errors: Identification and strategies to avoid frequent spelling mistakes.

Homophones and Homonyms: Clarification of words with similar auditory characteristics but differing meanings and spellings.

Abbreviations and Acronyms: Correct punctuation and spelling for abbreviated terms commonly encountered in healthcare settings.

By the conclusion of this chapter, you will possess a comprehensive understanding of punctuation and spelling, enabling you to excel in relevant portions of the ATI TEAS® Exam and to communicate more effectively in a professional healthcare context.

26.2 Essential Punctuation Marks: Commas, Periods, and Semicolons

Navigating the complex arena of punctuation necessitates focused attention. This section concentrates on three foundational punctuation marks that are both frequently employed and commonly misunderstood: commas, periods, and semicolons. These marks function as the linguistic traffic signals that orchestrate the reader's journey through your narrative.

Commas

The comma, diminutive yet potent, has the capacity to introduce a plethora of misunderstandings if misused. Its functions include separating items in a series, demarcating introductory phrases, and distinguishing independent clauses conjoined by coordinating conjunctions such as "and," "but," or "so." Examples include:

Items in a series: "I purchased apples, bananas, and grapes."

Introductory elements: "Nevertheless, she disagreed with the decision."

Independent clauses: "She was fatigued, yet she completed her work."

Periods

The period serves as the terminal punctuation mark, indicating the completion of a fully-formed thought. Despite its apparent simplicity, its strategic placement is crucial for preserving the intended meaning and coherence of a sentence.

Semicolons

Semicolons function as an intermediate punctuation mark, bridging closely related independent clauses or separating items in lists that already include commas. They offer a softer pause than periods but a stronger syntactical connection than commas.

26.3 Addressing Common Spelling Errors: Homophones and Silent Letters

Spelling constitutes a crucial facet of written communication. While automated spellcheck tools offer valuable assistance, they are not foolproof. This segment addresses two frequent sources of spelling errors: homophones and silent letters.

Homophones

Homophones are words that, despite sharing auditory similarities, differ in meaning and spelling. Errors involving homophones often escape automated spellcheck tools, necessitating extra caution during manual proofreading.

Silent Letters

Silent letters present another challenge, originating from the word's etymological background. Mastery of these idiosyncrasies is achieved through consistent practice and rote memorization.

Concluding Remarks

The intricacies of spelling and punctuation may appear daunting, but they are surmountable through diligent practice. Gaining proficiency in these areas will augment not only your performance on standardized tests like the ATI TEAS® Exam but also your efficacy in professional written communication.

Part VII: Test Day Tips

Chapter 27: Preparing for Test Day

27.1 Introduction to Test Day Preparedness

The Assessment Technologies Institute Test of Essential Academic Skills (ATI TEAS®) Exam is an imperative juncture in your pursuit of a career in healthcare. While academic preparation is undeniably important, logistical and emotional readiness should not be overlooked. This chapter is designed to furnish you with essential strategies to optimize focus and mitigate stress on test day. The most meticulously prepared candidates may falter if the significance of comprehensive test day preparation is underestimated.

The Imperative of Comprehensive Test Day Preparedness

The axiom, "Failure to prepare is preparing to fail," is particularly pertinent when approaching high-stakes assessments like the ATI TEAS®. This exam not only measures your academic acumen but also evaluates your aptitude for time management and stress regulation—skills indispensable to the healthcare field. A holistic preparation approach should incorporate academic mastery as well as practical and emotional readiness.

Chapter Overview

This chapter will address a multitude of factors to ensure your effective test day preparation, including:

Essential and prohibited items for the test center

Strategies for managing test-induced anxiety

Time management protocols specific to the test day

Techniques for sustained focus and endurance throughout the exam

By delving into these facets, we aspire to offer an exhaustive guide to navigate test day successfully. Let us begin our preparation for this pivotal milestone in your professional journey.

Significance of a Test Day Routine

The establishment of a well-calibrated test day routine can be transformative. This encompasses activities not just on the morning of the exam, but also in the preceding days. A judiciously planned routine can:

Synchronize your physiological and psychological rhythms to the test schedule

Anticipate and neutralize potential distractors

Cultivate a comfort level that minimizes test-related anxiety

For instance, if your test is scheduled for 9:00 a.m., consider adhering to the same wake-up time you intend for the test day. Incorporate a balanced breakfast, a concise review session, and potentially light exercise to activate your circulation. The objective is to normalize the conditions of test day.

Conclusion

Preparation for test day is not merely ancillary; it is integral to your comprehensive ATI TEAS® Exam strategy. The forthcoming sections will elaborate on each dimension of test day preparedness, offering actionable insights to enhance your performance. Stay engaged as we strive to make your test day a triumph.

27.2 Test Day Checklist

Your long-awaited test day has arrived, and it's time to deploy your accumulated knowledge in the ATI TEAS® Exam. Before you step out, it is vital to confirm that you are well-equipped for a seamless testing experience. This section provides an extensive checklist for test day, categorized into essential items to carry and items to avoid.

Items to Carry

Identification: A valid photo ID, such as a driver's license or passport, is indispensable. Ensure its validity and name-match with your test registration.

Admission Ticket: Secure a printout or digital copy of your admission ticket, displaying essential test center details.

Writing Implements: Carry a minimum of two sharpened pencils with erasers and an ink pen for form completion.

Time-keeping Device: Though test centers usually feature wall clocks, a simple wristwatch is advisable for personal time tracking.

Nutritional Supplies: Pack light snacks and water to maintain energy levels during your test center tenure.

Adaptive Clothing: Given variable test center temperatures, layered attire is recommended for comfort adjustment.

Positive Disposition: Above all, bring along a sense of confidence and optimism. Your preparation has equipped you for this.

Items to Avoid

Electronic Gadgets: Refrain from carrying cell phones, calculators, or other electronic devices, as they are typically disallowed.

Study Materials: Leave behind notes, textbooks, and other academic aids; they are generally prohibited.

Oversized Bags: Opt for compact bags that can be easily stowed, as large bags are often restricted.

Noise-Inducing Items: Avoid carrying items like keys or loose change that could disrupt the testing environment.

Unapproved Food and Beverages: While basic snacks are usually acceptable, noisy or distracting items should be avoided.

Negative Mindset: Discard any residual doubts or anxieties before entering the test center.

By adhering to this checklist, you are optimally positioning yourself for a successful and unencumbered test day experience. Be sure to review this list meticulously before departure, ensuring your preparedness for the ATI TEAS® Exam.

27.3 Psychological Preparedness: Stress Management Techniques

Your material preparations may be in place, but what about your psychological readiness? Test days can indeed be fraught with tension, making stress management critical for peak performance. This section explores various strategies for stress alleviation and psychological well-being.

Deep Breathing Techniques

A simple yet effective mechanism for stress modulation is deep breathing. Prioritize this practice to enhance oxygenation and consequently reduce stress levels before the test.

Visualization Strategies

Mental imagery, envisioning your smooth progression through the exam and satisfactory completion, can be a potent tool for both stress reduction and self-confidence enhancement.

Progressive Muscle Relaxation

If muscle tension is an issue, consider progressive muscle relaxation. This entails the sequential tensing and relaxing of muscle groups, culminating in a state of overall physical relaxation.

Positive Affirmations

Verbal affirmations like "I am prepared" or "I am capable" can significantly shift your psychological stance from one of anxiety to one of readiness and competence.

Mindfulness and Grounding Exercises

Utilize grounding techniques, such as the 5-4-3-2-1 method, to refocus attention during moments of distraction or heightened stress.

Scheduled Breaks and Physical Movements

Brief intermissions for stretching or shifting your gaze can serve as mental resets, bolstering your focus and attention.

Psychological readiness is as crucial as academic preparedness. By integrating these stress management techniques into your test day regimen, you bolster your capacity to manage the rigors of the ATI TEAS® Exam effectively. Maintain your composure; you are well-prepared for this challenge.

Chapter 28: Strategies for Test-Taking

28.1 The Significance of Strategic Planning

You have invested significant effort into your preparation, but your readiness is not solely dependent on your familiarity with the subject matter. A robust strategic approach is also vital for optimal performance during the examination. A well-considered strategy can effectively assist in time management, prioritizing questions, and enhancing your overall confidence. The importance of a planned approach is analogous to a military strategy: one does not enter a battlefield without a tactical plan. A strong strategy enables you to maximize your ability to display your knowledge comprehensively during the examination.

<u>Scope of Topics Covered</u>

In this chapter, we will focus on a range of test-taking methodologies that are specifically designed for the ATI TEAS® Exam. The strategies will equip you to confront diverse question types, including multiple-choice, fill-in-the-blank, and the more complex true/false queries. We will investigate techniques for improving reading comprehension, interpreting data, and will also offer guidance for excelling in the science and mathematics sections. Additional topics will include how to approach uncertain questions and the conditions under which guessing might be advantageous.

Our discussion extends beyond mere accuracy in responding to questions; it is about optimizing your entire test-taking experience. This involves the careful reading of questions, effective elimination of incorrect options, and the efficient management of time.

In summary, this chapter aspires to provide a comprehensive toolkit of tactics to streamline your test-taking experience, enhancing both efficiency and success. Let us proceed to delve into the detailed strategies tailored for the ATI TEAS® Exam.

28.2 Time Management: Test Pacing and Scheduled Breaks

<u>Time Allocation</u>

Effective time management is critical in an exam setting. A common impediment often faced by test-takers is inadequate pacing, which may result in hurried responses or unanswered questions. To preclude this, a pacing strategy should be devised prior to the examination. Familiarize yourself with the total time allocated and the volume of questions to be answered. Calculate an average time-per-question to guide your pacing.

However, this is not a one-size-fits-all approach. Some questions may demand more focused attention and time, while others may be dispatched quickly. Flexibility is key; it is advisable to continuously monitor your time. If confronted with a particularly challenging question, mark it for review and proceed, revisiting it later if time permits.

Scheduled Intermissions

Examinations like the ATI TEAS® are akin to a marathon rather than a sprint. Recognizing when to take brief mental recesses is crucial for maintaining focus. While some exams have pre-specified breaks, micro-breaks can also be personally instituted. These are momentary pauses for relaxation and cognitive resetting before reengaging with the test.

Utilize scheduled breaks for stretching, hydration, and perhaps a quick snack. Refrain from reviewing notes or engaging in last-minute cramming, as it can induce stress and is unlikely to be beneficial at this juncture. The objective is to return to the test invigorated and focused.

In conclusion, mastering both pacing and scheduled breaks constitutes effective time management. This combination enables you to allocate time judiciously among questions and to refresh and refocus when needed, optimizing your overall performance.

28.3 The Strategy of Elimination

Multiple-choice questions offer both opportunity and risk. While the correct response is among the available options, so are distractors—deceptively incorrect choices designed to mislead. Employing elimination techniques enhances your likelihood of selecting the correct answer. Carefully read each question and assess the relevance and accuracy of each answer choice in relation to it. Options containing absolutes, such as "always" or "never," are generally red flags indicative of distractors, as are overly complex or extraneous options.

The Value of Educated Guessing

Upon eliminating implausible options, you are left with "educated guesses." These are choices made based on a higher probability of accuracy. Sometimes you might be left with only two choices, thus significantly increasing your odds of being correct.

It is crucial to remember that an educated guess is preferable to an unanswered question, especially in exams like the ATI TEAS®, which do not penalize for incorrect answers. Employing this technique is particularly useful in time-sensitive sections of the test.

To summarize, the art of elimination significantly improves your test-taking strategy. It provides a structured approach to navigate the complexity of multiple-choice questions, enhances your confidence, and maximizes your time efficiency. Coupled with other strategies like time management, this skill can substantially improve your performance on the ATI TEAS® Exam.

Chapter 29: Post-Examination Analysis

29.1 The Significance of Reflective Assessment

Post-Examination Reflection: A Strategic Imperative

Completing the ATI TEAS® Exam may initially elicit a sense of relief, urging you to distance yourself from the experience as swiftly as possible. Although this sentiment is understandable, it is imperative to allocate time for reflective assessment. This practice is not a mere indulgence but serves as a cornerstone for your future academic and professional development.

Engaging in reflection enables a nuanced evaluation of your performance, delineating both your strong suits and areas necessitating further refinement. Were there challenges with time management? Were particular subject matters more difficult? Identifying these components will inform your strategies for forthcoming examinations and subsequent career or educational milestones.

Transforming Reflection into Constructive Insights

Reflection transcends mere contemplation; it is an avenue for deriving actionable strategies. After identifying areas of improvement, you can customize your study plan accordingly. Whether you encountered issues with time management or specific subject areas, tailored approaches such as additional timed questions, practice tests, or expert consultation can help augment your understanding.

Furthermore, reflection is not singularly focused on weaknesses; it also entails acknowledging your strengths. Did you excel in specific topics like algebra or reading comprehension? Recognizing your assets can heighten your self-assurance and serve as a strategic advantage in future assessments.

Reflective practice also contributes to emotional resilience. It furnishes a sense of closure to the stressful pre-examination phase and reconciles your expectations with actual performance. This emotional catharsis is integral for mental health and readies you for ensuing challenges.

In summary, reflection is an active, forward-looking endeavor that enriches your future preparedness based on experiential learning and individual insights.

29.2 Evaluation of Performance Metrics

<u>Methods to Access Test Scores</u>

Post-examination, you may wonder, "What was my performance?" While the ATI TEAS® Exam doesn't offer immediate score access, it furnishes a systematic approach to obtain your results. Typically available within a few days to a week, these scores can be accessed via ATI Testing's online portal using your registration credentials.

It is crucial to adhere to the particular guidelines set by the administering institution, as they may have distinct procedures for score distribution, ranging from printed copies to email notifications.

<u>Interpreting Your Score Report</u>

Upon retrieving your scores, the report might initially appear complex, replete with numerical data and terminology. This report is organized into distinct sections correlating to the tested subjects—Reading, Mathematics, Science, and English and Language Usage. It generally features both raw scores and percentile ranks, the latter offering a comparative measure of your performance.

Beyond mere numerical indicators, the score report serves as a roadmap for future action plans. Low scores in specific sections can highlight areas requiring attention, while high scores can validate the efficacy of your preparation methods.

29.3 Strategies for Future Endeavors or Retakes

<u>Effective Study Techniques for Enhancement</u>

Post-examination, the subsequent steps are integral to your academic trajectory. If a retake is warranted, consider this an opportunity for focused improvement. Utilize the score report to pinpoint your weaker areas, then adapt your study plans to address these deficiencies using an array of resources.

Should your scores meet or exceed your program's criteria, leverage your strong areas to cultivate deeper subject matter expertise. The ATI TEAS® Exam is but one milestone; performing commendably should propel further academic pursuits.

Universal Study Techniques

Regardless of your next steps, several effective study methods are universally beneficial:

Active Recall and Spaced Repetition: Utilize techniques backed by empirical evidence to optimize your study sessions.

Practice Tests: Simulate examination conditions to refine time management skills.

Peer-Led Study Sessions: Collaborative learning can provide diverse perspectives and facilitate a better grasp of challenging concepts.

Holistic Well-Being: A balanced diet, sufficient rest, and physical exercise can substantially impact cognitive performance.

Mindfulness Techniques: Employ relaxation methods to mitigate stress, thereby enhancing focus and test performance.

In conclusion, the period following the ATI TEAS® Exam should not be underestimated; it is an opportunity for continuous improvement or academic progression. The actionable insights derived from your performance are invaluable for future endeavors.

Conclusion: A Reflective Summary

As we conclude this comprehensive guide, it is imperative to contemplate the transformative journey upon which you are embarking. Preparing for the ATI TEAS® Exam transcends mere factual memorization and mastery of test-taking techniques; it establishes the foundation for your forthcoming career in healthcare. While the road ahead will undoubtedly present challenges, it is prudent to view each obstacle as a veiled opportunity for growth.

The Imperative of Perseverance

Foremost, it is essential to acknowledge the indispensable role of perseverance. Whether you are undertaking the exam for the initial or subsequent times, your unyielding resolve to succeed serves as your most powerful asset. The trajectory toward success is often punctuated by setbacks, yet these should not be construed as termini. Rather, they function as instructive detours that enrich your journey towards your ultimate objectives.

The Significance of Self-Efficacy

Equally critical is the concept of self-efficacy. Your confidence in your abilities can substantially influence your performance outcomes. Negative self-perceptions and uncertainties can obfuscate your clarity of thought and impair your concentration. Counteract these tendencies through the adoption of affirmative self-talk and positive visualizations. Envision yourself excelling in the exam and receiving the coveted acceptance letter from your ideal academic program, and allow these projections to invigorate your preparatory efforts.

The Contribution of Support Networks

The value of a robust support network cannot be underestimated. Be it family, friends, or mentors, a circle of individuals who have faith in your abilities can have a transformative impact. Share your aspirations and apprehensions with these confidants, seek their counsel, and allow their affirmations to elevate your spirits. Often, a mere handful of encouraging words can convert an unproductive study session into a fruitful endeavor.

The Necessity of Effective Time Management

Effective time management is a skill that will find utility not only in your immediate academic preparations but also in your future professional life. Cultivating the ability to prioritize tasks, allocate time judiciously, and schedule constructive intermissions are habits that will benefit you indefinitely. Employ organizational tools such as digital planners, mobile applications, or traditional task lists to monitor your academic regimen.

The Role of Comprehensive Well-Being

Prioritize your physical and mental well-being alongside your academic commitments. Engage in regular physical exercise, maintain a balanced dietary regimen, and ensure sufficient rest. Incorporate stress-reduction techniques, including meditation and diaphragmatic breathing exercises, to preserve a tranquil disposition, particularly valuable during the examination.

The Continuum of Lifelong Learning

It is pivotal to recognize that the ATI TEAS® Exam constitutes merely a single juncture in your enduring educational odyssey. Whether you excel or necessitate a retake, each experience confers invaluable insights. The proficiencies you cultivate—such as discipline, time management, and critical thinking—are not confined to test-specific applications; they are transferable life skills.

The Final Stage

As the examination day looms, it is typical to experience a confluence of anticipation and trepidation. This pivotal moment has been the focus of your preparatory efforts, and its realization is imminent. Have faith in your preparatory rigor, maintain confidence in your capabilities, and deliver your optimum performance. Upon conclusion, irrespective of the outcome, allocate a moment for self-recognition and appreciation of your committed exertions.

The Subsequent Chapter

Whether your result necessitates advancement or reevaluation, understand that this is merely the inaugural phase of your broader journey within the healthcare sector—a sector that uniquely affords the privilege of substantially impacting lives.

In summary, may the following affirmation guide you: "I possess the capability, exhibit resilience, and am incrementally advancing toward my aspirations." With this resolute mindset, no challenge is insurmountable, and no objective remains unattainable. We extend our most heartfelt wishes for success in your ATI TEAS® Exam and the promising future that inevitably lies beyond.

EXERCISES AND EXTRA CONTENT

1) **3000 QUESTIONS AND ASWERS (500 MATHS, 1000 USE OF LANGUAGE, 1500 SCIENCE)**

2) **308 TEACHING CARDS (USE OF LANGUAGE, CHEMISTRY, MATHEMATICS, ANATOMY AND BIOLOGY)**

3) **N. 3 TEST SIMULATIONS**

Made in the USA
Middletown, DE
11 September 2024

60726394R00051